PRIMARY HEALTH CARE OF THE WELL ADULT

D1479794

PRIMARY HEALTH CARE OF THE WELL ADULT

NANCY DIEKELMANN, R.N., M.S.

Assistant Professor
Primary Health Care Division
University of Wisconsin
School of Nursing

McGraw-Hill Book Company
A BLAKISTON PUBLICATION

New York   St. Louis   San Francisco   Auckland
Bogotá   Düsseldorf   Johannesburg   London
Madrid   Mexico   Montreal   New Delhi
Panama   Paris   São Paulo   Singapore
Sydney   Tokyo   Toronto

NOTICE

Medicine is an ever-changing science. As new research and clinical experience broaden our knowledge, changes in treatment and drug therapy are required. The editors and the publisher of this work have made every effort to ensure that the drug dosage schedules herein are accurate and in accord with the standards accepted at the time of publication. Readers are advised, however, to check the product information sheet included in the package of each drug they plan to administer to be certain that changes have not been made in the recommended dose or in the contraindications for administration. This recommendation is of particular importance in regard to new or infrequently used drugs.

This book was set in Century Medium by Allen Wayne Technical Corp.
The editors were Sally J. Barhydt and Michael Gardner;
the designer was Joan E. O'Connor;
the production supervisor was Robert C. Pedersen.
The cover was designed by Ruth Reis.
R. R. Donnelley & Sons Company was printer and binder.

PRIMARY HEALTH CARE OF THE WELL ADULT

1234567890 DODO 783210987

Library of Congress Cataloging in Publication Data

Diekelmann, Nancy.
    Primary health care of the well adult.

    "A Blakiston publication."
    Includes index.
    1. Hygiene. 2. Nursing. 3. Medicine, Preventive.
I. Title. [DNLM: 1. Primary health care—Nursing
texts. 2. Nurse-Patient relations. 3. Patients—
Education—Nursing texts. WY87 D559p]
RT67.D53   613′.02′4613   76-46868
ISBN 0-07-016879-2

TO JOHN
FOR HIS PATIENCE
AND LOVE

Contents

Preface

"I'm twenty-one! Should I really only be eating three eggs a week?"

"Are adults supposed to receive immunizations?"

"I've heard that cancer runs in families. My father just had surgery for lung cancer. I guess I really shouldn't be smoking, should I?"

Nurses are asked questions like these by patients in a variety of settings, from physicians' offices to bedside situations. It is our role as nurses to provide for patient education, but too often the information we offer focuses on disease or disease prevention rather than on health maintenance and health promotion.

As growing attention is given to primary health care, it is more important than ever that nurses provide patient education in health maintenance and health promotion, whether they find themselves in a primary or secondary health care setting. The office nurse can use the time that patients spend waiting to see the doctor to talk about adult needs for immunizations. While making a middle-aged woman's bed, the hospital nurse can initiate a discussion about menopause and the changes related to it.

Such teaching and counseling requires a knowledge of normal or *well* adults, their health care needs, and nursing interventions to meet those needs. Such information is both scarce and scattered. Data related to the normal adult comes from many fields, from normal nutrition to human population ecology. Few nurses have the time to assemble it and frequently such data are not a part of our disease-oriented nursing curricula. Consequently, clients and patients often go without this useful information.

This book is meant to help correct some of our shortcomings by focusing on the assessment of the primary health care needs of the well adult, rather than dealing in any detail with the physical assessment—history and physical examination. It will offer situations and interventions and include vignettes of patient-nurse interactions to help students and nurses apply their knowledge of the adult assessment and primary health care to the nursing care they are providing in both primary and secondary settings.

ACKNOWLEDGMENTS

The author appreciates the support and assistance received from many friends. I am especially grateful to Ednah Shepard Thomas for her valuable help in preparing the manuscript, and to Sally Barhydt and Michael Gardner of McGraw-Hill for their valuable guidance.

I am especially indebted to Sheila E. Dresen for her contributions of writing the chapters on sexuality and menopause. She also provided valuable insight and support during all phases of preparing this manuscript.

In addition, the following persons are acknowledged for reviewing the manuscript, partially or in total: Bernard B. Wolfberg, M.D., Associate Director, Katharine Wright Psychiatric Clinic; Donald A. West, Assistant Clinical Professor of Psychiatry, University of New Mexico; Jonna Guendling, R.N., M.S.; and Signe S. Cooper, Professor and Chairman, University of Wisconsin Extension.

Also, for their help in researching this book, thank you to my special friends, Megan Hudson, Linda Johnson, and Loretta Hitzman.

And to Valencia N. Prock, Dean and Professor, School of Nursing, University of Wisconsin, Madison, for her support and leadership in the development of primary health care, go many thanks.

Nancy Diekelmann

PRIMARY HEALTH CARE OF THE WELL ADULT

Living Sensibly

The Young Adult

PART ONE

CHAPTER 1

Young Adulthood– An Overview

There are a variety of changes occurring in today's society that are influencing the early years of the young adult. Marriage has lost its permanence, and the divorce rate is soaring. The availability of abortion offers options not present before, as does the availability of day-care centers. Increasingly, women seek equality and fulfillment beyond the home. For 1975, *Time* magazine presented no Man of the Year, but instead twelve Women of the Year. It is no longer taken for granted that the wife and mother will stay home; in fact, it is almost taken for granted that she will not. She may work outside the home because the family needs the money, which is increasingly true as living costs steadily rise, or she may work outside for self-fulfillment. She may, of course, work outside for both reasons. The American family pattern today is a blurred one, in a state of constant flux. The woman may be isolated from the home, spending much of her waking time in a job or a profession. The man may see much more of his children than ever before and receive new satisfaction in helping with the child-rearing aspect of the family. This in turn may lead to the male's domestication and children who grow up to condemn and reject materialistic values. Change is constant.

CHANGE AND HEALTH

We live in a period so marked by continuous and far-reaching changes that we accept change as the normal way of life. Recently, research has shown the significance that change has on the health of an individual.[1] It appears that the quantity of life change and the degree to which one's life-style is altered by this change have been shown to have an effect on physiological adaptation.

> It has been established that "alterations of life style" which require a great deal of adjustment and coping correlate with illness—whether or not these changes are under the individual's own direct control, and whether or not he sees them as undesirable. Furthermore, the higher the risk that subsequent illness will be severe. So strong is the evidence that it is becoming possible, by studying life change scores, actually to predict levels of illness in various populations.[2]

T. H. Holmes has devised a scale that assigns point values to changes that often affect human beings. When enough of these changes occur within 1 year and their point values add up to more than 300, illness may lie ahead. In Holmes' survey, 80 percent of people whose point values exceeded 300 became pathologically depressed, had heart attacks, or developed other serious ailments. Fifty-three percent of those who scored in the 150 to 300 range were similarly affected, as were 33 percent of those scoring up to 150.[3] (See Table 1-1.)

VIGNETTE

Emory was married. Soon, as he had hoped, his wife became pregnant and stopped working. She gave birth to a healthy baby girl. After the baby was born, Emory changed jobs. He found a better paying job by changing his line of work and went into administration. After a short vacation, he moved his family to the suburbs, returned to hunting, which he had so enjoyed as an adolescent, and began making new friends by socializing with his new colleagues. He felt so good about everything that was happening to him, that he even stopped smoking!

In our example, Emory's marriage (50), his wife's pregnancy (40), her stopping work (26) and bearing a daughter (39), changing jobs (38), to a different line of work (36), his vacation (13), their move to the suburbs (20), change in recreation (18), and giving up smoking (24) all total 323. Thus Emory is a candidate for developing a depression or some other serious illness. While the full extent to which this information can be utilized in a preventative approach is not known, Holmes claims that one of the ways physical and emotional illness can be prevented is through counseling susceptible people not to effect too many life changes in too short a time.

TABLE 1-1

Life Event	Value
Death of spouse	100
Divorce	73
Marital separation	65
Jail term	63
Death of close family member	63
Personal injury or illness	53
Marriage	50
Fired at work	47
Marital reconciliation	45
Retirement	45
Change in health of family member	44
Pregnancy	40
Sex difficulties	39
Gain of new family	39
Change in financial state	38
Death of close friend	37
Change to different line of work	36
Change in number of arguments with spouse	35
Mortgage over $10,000	31
Foreclosure of mortgage or loan	30
Change in responsibilities at work	29
Son or daughter leaving home	29
Trouble with in-laws	29
Outstanding personal achievement	28
Wife beginning or stopping work	26
Beginning or ending school	26
Revision of personal habits	24
Trouble with boss	23
Change in work hours or conditions	20
Change in residence	20
Change in schools	20
Change in recreation	19
Change in social activities	18
Mortgage or loan less than $10,000	17
Change in sleeping habits	16
Change in number of family get-togethers	15
Change in eating habits	15
Vacation	13
Minor violations of the law	11

PHYSIOLOGICAL CHANGES OF THE YOUNG ADULT

Completion of physical maturation occurs early in young adulthood. The systems of the body are functioning at their peak effectiveness. The young adult, age 20 to 39, has reached optimum mental and motor functions. Posture is erect and the skin is smooth. Cell multiplication and tissue repair is unimpaired. At the age of 20 the circulatory system is fully developed.

Aging begins at 20, though it will take another decade before most of the signs are perceptible and wrinkles and gray hair can be observed. The cardiovascular system, however, begins to show the signs of aging before the other systems. Hypertension and related cardiac problems, including silent heart disease, can be found in young adults now with increasing rapidity, and nurses should encourage young adults in their early twenties to have an electrocardiogram (ECG) as a baseline to monitor potential cardiovascular changes.

EMOTIONAL CHANGES OF THE YOUNG ADULT

Since research seems to indicate that change rather than stress may serve to precipitate a health crisis, the primary health care nurse needs to assess change in all areas. F. J. Duhl has outlined five types of emotional changes that commonly occur.[4]

The first is *change in an individual's view of his psychological self.* A worker may fail to get an expected promotion. A parent whose attention has been distracted may feel guilty because the unwatched child got hurt—fell off a windowsill, knocked over a boiling tea kettle, or ran into the path of a car.

The second is a *change in belief, values, and expectations.* This change is ideological and frequently involves areas of religion, politics, and sexual behavior. It can be an area that is full of many stressors for the young adult. The third change involves *changes in the relevant social network;* these changes occur in separation, divorce, the death of a friend or loved one, or the addition of a new child to the family. A *change in the nonhuman environment,* such as getting a new car or moving to a new home and leaving behind the old with its associations, is the fourth change. A *change in body image or the physical self* is the fifth change. Young adults are particularly sensitive about their appearance, and the addition of a few extra pounds or new glasses may be embarrassing to them. A real change in body image, such as an amputation or plastic surgery is, of course, very threatening.

DEVELOPMENTAL MILESTONES OF THE YOUNG ADULT

Transadulthood It has been customary to consider the age period from 20 to 40 as a whole, but it would seem now that a new stage is developing in its early part—very largely as a result of social factors. Carl Danzinger and Matthew Greenwald, sociologists from Rutgers University, have given this period the name *transadulthood.* It is interesting that the term "adolescent" was not coined until 1904, when, with compulsory high school education and the resulting extended stay in school, teenagers began to be identified as a specific group. A similar phenomenon is to be observed today. The demand and opportunity for education are so much greater that many more years are now devoted to it, with the result of the postponement of a job and often of marriage. Today it would be unthinkable to call an unmarried woman of 25 an "old maid," and it is taken as a matter of course that many a man of 26 has never worked at his profession, but is still engaged in his graduate work or medical or legal training. We might say, perhaps, that transadults have 10 more years, those from 20 to 30, to "group up" in than was the case with their counterparts a generation ago.

The growing up does not always proceed very smoothly. For one thing, since it is a new phenomenon, there are no models and precedents which help young people to meet it. Transadults are sexually and intellectually mature, but not necessarily emotionally mature, as yet unemployed, without the sobering responsibility of parenthood, and generally, particularly among the affluent, with a good deal of leisure time. Many have become very much involved in social and political movements, particularly in the period of the Vietnam war. They are more or less forced to rely on their own resources to become adults. "They must develop appropriate styles of behavior for which there are no parental models."[5]

With our rapid rate of change, life-styles are multiplying. So are a variety of occupations, and a high degree of specialization is developing within them. A teacher may be a specialist in the field of audiovisual arts, and an electrician may be trained to work only in industrial settings. More opportunities than ever before are open to women. The very range of choice is in itself a difficult problem. The schools are at a loss as to what to teach which will be valid and useful by the time their students graduate, and how to better prepare them for the world they will be living in, a world which will be very different from the present one. How, indeed, will the nurse herself be adequately prepared for the future?

Many observers of the transadults, particularly those closely involved, like parents, may worry that they will never reenter the mainstream of society. Carl Danziger and Matthew Greenwald, however, feel they are likely to do so at about the age of 30. It is of course too early to document this phenomenon statistically, but there seems to be evidence that about then there is a general tendency to settle down. A typical transadult couple have been living together for some time. More and more of their friends are getting married.

They think they may as well do so themselves. They start work. They save enough money to buy a little economy car. From then on, they never look back. They have become young adults.

Some adolescents, specifically those who are not affluent and who belong to minority populations, may become adult without going through the transadult phase. Ghetto adolescents are very limited in the variety of people they meet from other various socioeconomic classes, national origins, or educational backgrounds. They have no opportunity to enjoy early dating that is marked by picnics and proms. In the ghetto, one hand may have to be held in the pocket on a knife; a picnic in the park would be an invitation to robbery, or worse. Thus in the ghettos there is virtually no engagement period, and dating leads quickly to physical involvement and sometimes to pregnancy and early parenthood, often with no marriage or spouse. In order to survive, some couples are forced to take on responsibility very early. Generally both husband and wife or the single parent must work. If either loses a job, they may have to move in with parents, which may well mean overcrowding, lack of privacy, and conflict. Of necessity, then, there is no transition period for these adolescents; they are thrust immediately into young adulthood.

The Thirties Studies are currently being conducted to further identify the phases of adult life. According to a Yale study (involving only men), at about age 30 to 35, the male goes through a settling down period.[6] The individual makes deeper commitments, invests more of himself in his work, family, and valued interests and, within the framework of this life structure, makes and pursues more long-range plans and goals. He begins to "settle down" in that he finds his niche, builds a nest, and pursues his interests. However, he also is concerned with "making it." This involves planning, striving, and upward mobility.

The next stage, which occurs during the years from age 35 to 39, focuses on becoming one's "own man." It is during this period that no matter what the man has accomplished to date, he feels not sufficiently his own man. This sense of constraint and oppression may occur not only in work but also in marriage and other relationships. During this period, the man may develop a relationship with a mentor, a man usually 8 to 15 years older than himself. The mentor is enough older to represent greater wisdom, authority, and paternal qualities, but near enough in age or attitudes to be in some respects a peer or older brother rather than the image of the wise old man or distant father. The mentor initiates the younger man into the new occupation and guides, criticizes, and encourages him for perhaps

3 or 4 years. Then a difference of opinion arises, separation occurs, and the younger man emerges into the forties on his own. This relationship enables the young man to interact as an adult with another man who regards him as an adult and who welcomes him into the adult world on a relatively (but not completely) mutual and equal basis. The young man must in time reject this relationship, largely because it has served its purpose.

Another study done by Dr. Gould at the University of California at Los Angeles attempts to describe and identify the phases of adult life by use of an intensive interviewing technique.[7] He discovered that between the ages of 29 and 34, questions such as "What is life all about now that I am doing what I am supposed to?" and "Is what I am the only way for me to be?" were common. He characterizes these young adults as weary of devoting themselves to the task of being what they are supposed to (although they continue on) and just want to be what they are. In the subsequent age group, ages 35 to 43, there is a continued look within and an existential questioning of self, values, and life itself, but with a change of tone toward quiet desperation and an increasing awareness of a time squeeze. Common statements were "I just want to be," "Have I done the right things?" and "Is there time to change?"

Unfortunately the developmental milestones of the young adult are not comprehensively articulated as they are for the infant and the toddler. But research is moving in that direction. Until then the nurse can generally only provide anticipatory guidance to the young adult.

DEVELOPMENTAL TASKS OF YOUNG ADULTS

VIGNETTE
Lora, who is 20 years old, lives with her parents and works for a local insurance company. At the clinic where she came for a prescription for birth control pills, she told the nurse who was taking her history that the fact that she had recently become a vegetarian was really bothering her parents. A few weeks ago, she continued, she had had a rash on her finger, but instead of going to the doctor as her mother told her to do, she treated it with some herbal cream given to her by a friend. "But look," she says, "It went away!"

In this period of change in the lives of young adults, there are four developmental tasks. As these developmental tasks are accomplished, young adults have new energy to continue their growth in other areas.

Establishing independence from their parents is the first of these tasks. This task is emotional, physical, and economic. The process of separation, of course, is lifelong; it begins at birth with the separation of the child from the mother, and ends only with death. Physically, it is well accomplished by the young adult moving out of the home and setting up housekeeping in the community. Economically and emotionally, it may be more difficult to separate and establish independence.

Economically, it is often difficult today for young adults to be independent of their parents, since now they spend many more years than was formerly the case in receiving their education; they therefore remain dependent on their parents for financial support, at least partially. (Sometimes students marry and the wife takes over the parents' role of supporting a husband who is finishing professional training.) If the young adult continues to live at home, he or she may have added difficulty in establishing certain rights of decision.

If young adults have jobs and their own living arrangements, they may reasonably feel economically independent of their parents. However, they may still be emotionally dependent if they keep in such close touch that they must report every little accomplishment, and if they continue to live "for" their parents with their parents' values and expectations of them as paramount. They may be afraid of making mistakes on their own, and so they seek out their parents' guidance rather than assuming responsibility and taking a chance on their own decision-making capabilities. Even after such a firm step toward independence as marriage, a man may take his wife regularly to have Sunday dinner with his parents. The wife may spend much time on the telephone through the week reporting trivial occurrences to her mother. Even when she has children of her own, though symbolically this act represents an even firmer assertion of independence, she may, ironically, grow dependent if she allows her mother too much active involvement.

The nurse can be helpful to young adults in the process of achieving independence by supporting a daughter the first time she does not return home to attend a cousin's wedding; or a son the first time he does not go home for Mother's Day but sends flowers and calls instead; or the couple who announce that they will celebrate Christmas Eve by themselves in their new apartment—together. Many times the young adult feels guilty when the parents misinterpret his behavior and view it as rejection and become angry with him. The nurse can provide anticipatory guidance by helping the young adult to anticipate the anger and rejection that might occur and to consider other alternatives.

For instance, the young couple who wish to celebrate Christmas Eve by themselves in their new apartment would inflict pain and invite anger if they did so while their parents were sitting at home neglected and alone, with nothing to do except remember all the past Christmas Eves which had been happy family occasions. However, the couple might consider whether other family members could be with the parents on the holiday; or they might suggest to the parents that they enter a new phase by sharing the evening with old friends whose children also were forming new ties elsewhere. A young man may have to discontinue the visit he has been in the habit of making home on Mother's Day; but he can send flowers or he can telephone. A young woman may not be able to afford either time or money to go back home for the wedding of a cousin; but she can send a present and let her mother know that she is genuinely interested in hearing all about the occasion.

Developing their own sense of values is the second developmental task for young adults. Typically they challenge the values of their parents and of society. Through challenging these values, the young adult is able to know which values of his parents he will alter, retain, or modify. Since values include religious, moral, and ethical issues, the questioning may be very painful to both the parents and the young adult. Sometimes this testing involves issues of sexuality, such as premarital sexual activity, and it can be very threatening to the parents who view this as a personal attack on their value system.

The nurse can help both the parents and the young adult by providing anticipatory guidance. She can show the parents that such questioning is normal and that it is essential since the young adult needs to have a sound basis on which to decide what values he will discard, modify, or retain. Young adults who leave their parents' form of worship may or may not return to it. The nurse can give the young adult an opportunity to discuss the implication of this type of testing and the reactions he may encounter in others when values generally held in society are challenged.

In the process of establishing independence from parents and in developing their own value systems, young adults may rebel against all forms of authority, not just their parents. This may include police officers, teachers, doctors, and indeed the nurse as well. If young adult clients are angry, aggressive, or defensive, the nurse should not react with her own aggressiveness or defensiveness. It is important that she be nonjudgmental. She needs to substantiate the reasons why and the implications of certain health behaviors and treatments to the young adult. She should clearly spell out the alternatives and then allow the young adult to select his own solution. The nurse should avoid, at all costs, any comments that sound like telling the young adult what to do.

Developing a sense of personal identity. The third developmental task is a particularly difficult one. This period is one of turmoil and frustration. Young adults begin to realize that each person is unique and they need to assert their individuality instead of becoming stereotypes such as "mother" or "salesperson."

Selecting a job or career is no longer a simple matter of inheriting the family farm. The bewildering number of possibilities in and out of the professions require many preliminary decisions about training. The present state of the American economy renders it extremely hard to select a job, since it is difficult to make a commitment without knowing if that job will be needed in another 10, 20, or 30 years.

Young adults establishing their working and family identities are beset by questions. Who am I? Who do I want to be? What do I care about? On what issues will I take a stand? The nurse aware of the importance of this task should be supportive.

Lastly, young adults must form intimate relationships with people outside the family. As the young adult separates from the family and begins establishing his own identity, there is now energy to be utilized in developing new adult relationships. This is a time of selecting mates, developing fewer but more intimate relationships with other young adults, starting a family, rearing children, and getting started in an occupation. This task involves a consideration of life-style and often a decision of whether or not to marry.

The nurse needs to recognize how important the peer group is at this time. If friends are smokers, for instance, a man or woman will find it especially hard to give up the habit. Young adults today live under a variety of conditions: in communes, in apartment complexes full of other young couples or singles, and in the suburbs. The norms of the peer group are important to the health behaviors of the young adult.

COPING WITH THE CHANGES OF YOUNG ADULTHOOD

A study has been made by Rachel Cox on sixty-three young men and women, whom she interviewed first as college undergraduates and then again 10 years later.[8] Although they all had made the transition into adulthood, the road had not always been a smooth one. She lists the following as the most frequently reported causes of conflict:

1 Shattered love affair
2 Career development slow or disappointing
3 Parents' marriage broken by divorce or marked by conflict
4 Harassed by indecision about whether vocational choice is good

5   Long-continued financial dependence on parents after college
6   Relation to mother too close emotionally, too dominated by her, or too distant
7   Neuroticism in parent
8   Relation to father too close emotionally, too dominated by him, or too distant
9   Financial stringency or insecurity in parental home

Confronted by these stress situations, young adults react in various ways. Many clients want assurance that their feelings are normal, and since "normal" is a difficult word to define, the nurse should encourage them to review their progress in achieving the previously mentioned developmental tasks. It may be helpful to encourage the young adult to seek outside help in resolving the stress situations in his life. The nurse should be prepared to offer a referral for further professional help.

Some young adults are very reluctant to seek such a service. One reason is the idea that you must be "crazy" if you are seeing a psychologist, psychiatric nurse, psychiatrist, or social worker. This view, of course, is pure myth. Probably no human being exists during these years of stress and strain who does not need the help of talking honestly and frankly to the right listener. Parents? Sometimes yes. But as Rachel Cox's list shows, often the problem is as much theirs as their children's. Furthermore, young adults engaged in the painful process of finding a solution are often reluctant to let their parents know how painful it is. Friends? Again, sometimes yes. The impulse to confide in a friend is common—as common as is regret at having done so. The professional listener is skilled and friendly and he will keep his mouth shut.

Another reason for their reluctance is expense. The nurse can help the young adult realize that problems can often be solved after only a few visits. Of course, much depends upon the type of problems involved and the goals of the young adult, but 50 minutes of a trained therapist's undivided attention can accomplish a great deal. A therapist can bring to the problem a fresh, unbiased view based on the perspective and knowledge derived from professional experience. He will suggest alternatives, and very importantly, he will provide sincere and interested support while the client selects an alternative and works out his own solution.

DEPRESSION

Depression, like the common cold, is an affliction to which we are all susceptible. It is sometimes the result of anger for which there is no outlet or no acceptable outlet. It is therefore turned against oneself and one becomes depressed. Sometimes young adults suppress their anger because they are afraid to let it out or because they think only children get angry. It's not easy to get angry at your boss or your teacher for fear of what they will do in return. At times, however, there is no one to blame or get angry at. At whom can one be angry for the death of a loved one? Depression can also occur as a reaction to a loss, such as a loss of close friends from college, death of parents or failure in getting a job that was anticipated. Young adults who understand the dynamics of depression may be able to find acceptable ways of expressing their anger, such as through physical exercise. Although depression does not necessarily lead to suicide any more than a cold necessarily leads to pneumonia, it may be a danger sign.

SUICIDE

Suicide is the third leading cause of death in the young adult,[9] and the nurse is frequently in a position to provide primary prevention. Primary prevention of suicide should include three areas. Early recognition of the suicidal young adult is of utmost importance. Whenever possible, the nurse should educate people about the advance signs of suicide, particularly those people who have the opportunity to come in contact with suicidal adults (people like students, faculty, and administrators). Secondly, there should be people available to the suicidal young adult who can offer a close relationship to compensate for a lost relationship or to provide the suicidal person with the help and concern he needs. This relationship can be provided by a counselor, psychiatrist, social worker, member of the clergy, psychiatric nurse, or psychologist. Lastly, young adults should be discouraged from leading lives of social isolation. The nurse should whenever possible encourage young adults to participate in outside activities to prevent social isolation. In order to function in these three areas, the primary health care nurse needs to know the latest information on suicide.

SUICIDE RESEARCH

Research has shown that it is possible to identify clients who may be a suicide risk.[12-13] Women make more suicide attempts than men, but men more often succeed; this is because women use less lethal methods, such as taking an overdose of aspirin or barbiturates or cutting the wrist, while men choose more lethal methods such as gunshot or hanging. According to statistics, suicide is least common among married persons, more common among single or widowed people, and most common among divorced persons. Professional groups such as dentists, psychiatrists, and other physicians are considered high risk. Young adults are more likely to *attempt* suicide than are older ones, but their methods are less lethal and therefore less likely to succeed. A suicide attempt can be simply a way of asking for help.

Events which commonly precipitate suicide usually involve serious interpersonal conflict: marital discord, family discord, loss of an intimate relationship, loss of personal resources, unemployment, or disappointment in work. Drinking heavily before a suicide attempt is common.[14]

Another symptom to observe is any sign of self-neglect. Clients may show decreased muscle tone, slumped shoulders, slowed gait and speech, and drooped facies. Lack of interest in work is significant, as is lack of interest in appearance. Finally, it is important to know of any previous suicide attempts. Suicide is 7 times more common among people who have made a previous attempt than among other depressed persons.[15]

Since suicide is the third leading cause of death among young adults, it is common in colleges and universities. Studies made in this setting show that those most likely to commit suicide are males who have average to above-average grades, come from middle-class families, are not satisfied with their present achievements, and spend much time alone. Suicide occurs more frequently among graduate than undergraduate students.[16]

Research has shown that the presuicidal state contains certain predictable behaviors:

1 Hypermobility
2 Reality testing impaired
3 High degree of helplessness and hopelessness expressed
4 Judgment and object relationships impaired
5 Less cooperative
6 Anorexia and weight loss
7 Increased pain threshold
8 Insomnia
9 Affect may be depressed, angry, bitter, or exhibiting fear or panic—few may feel happy, peaceful, and quiet[13]

When a nurse is concerned about a young adult, she may want to do a more thorough assessment.

Overt hostility, a history of overtly hostile relationships, a poor long-term work history, antisocial behavior, and a demanding and hostile current behavior may also indicate the potential for suicide.

The nurse should avoid becoming defensive with this client so the potential of suicide can be assessed. Some young adults attempt suicide as a gamble with death—a kind of Russian roulette. Research has shown that a majority of suicide attempts are characterized by risk-taking behavior. The implication of this research is that the nurse should never dare or challenge the young adult who may be forced to prove his sincerity or may be encouraged to risk the consequences of his behavior.[17]

VIGNETTE

Lavonia, a junior college student, comes in for her annual physical exam and tells the nurse that she is "having trouble with her stomach," has lost another 5 pounds, and wants some medication for constipation. She appears serious and she speaks slowly and in a monotone. The nurse pursues Lavonia's situation further. In the ensuing conversation, Lavonia tells the nurse that she is very concerned about her grade-point average. She is trying hard to bring it up to a B average, but she has one difficult course this semester and she may get a C. She says this is a good semester for her because she has moved out of the dorm and now lives by herself in a room with cooking privileges. She did this to save money, but she also has less distraction when she studies. She didn't go out for the girls' swimming team this semester because she wanted to devote all her attention to her studies. She talks about being frustrated with several of her teachers, but her facial appearance is one of anger—a feeling which she denies. After a few minutes of conversation with the nurse, she wants to see the doctor at once so she can have her physical and get something for her constipation. "I've got to get going," she says, "I have a lot of studying to do!"

The above vignette illustrates how a potentially suicidal patient may present herself to the nurse.

PRIMARY SUICIDE PREVENTION — THE ROLE OF THE NURSE

The nurse should be aware of the signs of suicide and should actively assess her clients. All remarks about suicide should be taken seriously. If a young adult speaks of helplessness or hopelessness or complains of feeling an emptiness to his life, the nurse should investigate further. She should be alert for signs of weight loss or gastrointestinal disturbances and sleep problems, as these complaints may indicate he is depressed. Depression is only one clue to potential suicide. The nurse should listen closely to the young adult if he speaks of feelings of alienation, of being unworthy of living, or of being in an impossible situation. He is a high-risk candidate.

If a client appears depressed, the nurse should not hesitate to ask the client if he has any suicidal thoughts, fantasies, or wishes.

Many nurses are afraid to talk to the depressed client about suicide for fear of putting ideas into the client's head. This is a myth.

The role of the primary health care nurse in suicide prevention varies from agency to agency. She needs to provide for education in the area of depression and its dynamics and prevention. Teaching the signs of a potential suicide is also important. But the nurse should also concern herself with the availability of outside activities to prevent social isolation in young adults. She also needs to be available and offer a supportive or therapeutic relationship to a suicidal young adult.

Obviously she needs to protect the client from his self-destructive impulses by seeing that he does not possess lethal weapons or potentially dangerous medication and that he give them up or dispose of them immediately. Emotional support is of great importance. The nurse needs to show that she understands and respects her client and that she sincerely cares about him. The nurse needs to be aware of her own feelings in this area. If she happens to be too depressed to be able to help her client, she should assume the responsibility for finding someone who can. If she has strong feelings about suicide, she can express them by saying, "I do not condone your choice of suicide as a way to solve your problem; but I can accept that at this point in time in your life, suicide may seem to you like the only way to deal with your problem." She may also add, "You may feel this way now, but you have no way of knowing how you will feel in a few days — especially with some help."

A number of suicide-prevention programs are currently in existence throughout the United States. These range from some manned a few hours a day by trained volunteers to 24-hour suicide-prevention phones located in psychiatric units, with trained professional personnel always available. The nurse should be aware of the resources in her community.

DIVORCE

Most divorces occur in the first 3 to 5 years of married life and involve persons under 29 years of age. These couples are often from lower economic groups and have married at an early age. They tend to have less education and money and fewer personal resources than couples from higher economic groups.[18]

Divorce is more common among persons poorly prepared for marriage, among those who marry to escape their parents, and among couples who cannot tolerate differences. It is also more common among children of divorced or unhappy parents, among childless marriages, and among pregnant brides.[19]

The percentage of persons divorced or separated is higher for black than for white persons and higher for women than for men.[20] There has been a significant increase in the divorce rate. This rate reflects national prosperity (when divorce increases) and a relaxation of social pressure against divorce. Statistics indicate that not only is the divorce rate higher, but there is a tendency of divorced persons to remain divorced (that is, to not remarry). However, according to Glick's study, about 75 percent of divorced persons remarry within 5 years and they marry other divorced individuals about 60 percent of the time.[21]

THE DIVORCE PROCESS

For a individual, divorce involves a process of resocialization and typically leads to rediscovering the art of dating and eventually to remarriage. After a divorce, the individual does not just shift from a married life back into a single life. Many things have changed and there is a need to reformulate a whole range of social ties from one's spouse and children to one's relatives and friends.

It is a time of ambivalent feeling: reactions of love and hate, mourning and relief, and feelings of failure and feelings of a new beginning. There are many difficult areas, such as sleeping alone, eating alone in restaurants (especially for men), and loneliness. During this time the divorced person may find a great deal of support from organizations such as Parents Without Partners or travel and ski clubs, but most particularly from divorced friends.

Dating is an important means of rediscovering one's value as a person and in repairing one's damaged ego and reestablishing moral-social ethics. But dating is more difficult for divorced persons, especially those with custody of small children. Children not only react to dating with a wide variety of feelings, but they also pose problems in terms of arrangements (babysitters, meals, and so on). Sexual relations are also more difficult if there are children in the home. (See Chapter 10, The Sexually Active Middle Adult.)

Remarriage will most likely be satisfactory when an individual enters into it with an understanding of how he has matured since his first marriage and of the reasons why his first marriage failed. However, if the mistakes of the first marriage are represented in finding a partner, the second marriage is also likely to fail. This person may meander from one relationship to another looking for satisfaction, yet the seeds of failure are within himself. Ideally, the second marriage should be entered into with time and thought.

DIVORCE AND THE YOUNG ADULT —
THE ROLE OF THE NURSE

Separated and divorced persons seem to be more vulnerable to mental and physical illness than married persons.[22] Their potential for having a health care crisis is high. The nurse can provide anticipatory guidance to young adults at this time by encouraging them to pay particular attention to their health needs.

The nurse is also in a position to recommend written materials that can help the young adult cope with the divorce. Since the legal aspects of the process of separation and divorce are often difficult and provide more chance for expressing anger than for smoothly facilitating divorce, there are now many materials available to help the individual better cope with all the legal aspects of divorce. The person will also need help with feelings of loss and guilt. The nurse can also help the parents anticipate the children's reactions to the divorce and the kind of behaviors to anticipate as the children accept the divorce. Children can be provided an opportunity to openly discuss some of their concerns during this very difficult transition. Lastly, the nurse should be aware of her own feelings about divorce and the divorced person.

BIBLIOGRAPHY

1* Sutterly, Doris Cook, and Gloria Ferraro Donnelly: *Perspectives in Human Development—Nursing Throughout the Life Cycle*, J. B. Lippincott Company, Philadelphia, 1973.

2 Toffler, A.: *Future Shock*, p. 293, Random House, Inc., New York, 1970.

3* Holmes, T. H., and R. H. Rahe: "The Social Readjustment Rating Scale," *J. Psychosom. Res.*, 2: 213-218, 1967.

4 Duhl, F. J.: "Grief," Paper presented to the Ohio League for Nursing Convention, Columbus, Ohio, 1964.

5* Mead, Margaret: *Culture and Commitment: A Study of the Generation Gap*, p. 46, Doubleday & Company, Inc., Garden City, N. Y., 1970.

6 Levinson, Daniel J., Charlotte N. Darrow, Edward B. Klein, Maria A. Levinson, and Braxton Mckee: "The Psychosocial Development of Men in Early Adulthood and the Mid-Life Transition," research report of the Research Unit for Social Psychology and Psychiatry, Connecticut Mental Health Center and the Department of Psychiatry, Yale University, 1972.

7 Gould, Roger L.: "The Phases of Adult Life: A Study in Developmental Psychology," *Am. J. Psychiat.* 129 (5): 33-43, 1972.

8 Cox, Rachel Dunaway: *Youth Into Maturity: A Study of Men and Women in the First Ten Years After College*, Mental Health Materials Center, New York, 1970.

9   Bahra, Robert J.: "The Potential for Suicide," *Am. J. Nursing*, 75 (10): 1782-1788, 1975.

10   Lester, Gene, and David Lester: *Suicide: The Gamble With Death*, Prentice-Hall, Inc., Englewood Cliffs, N. J., 1971.

11   Murphy, G. E.: "Clinical Identification of Suicidal Risk," *Arch. Gen. Psychiat.*, 27: 356-359, 1972.

12* Niccolini, R.: "Reading the Signals for Suicide Risks," *Geriatrics*, 28: 71-72, 1973.

13   "The Suicide Profile," *Brit. Med. J.*, 2: 525-526, 1975.

14   Mayfield, D. G., et al.: "Alcoholism, Alcohol Intoxication, and Suicide Attempts," *Arch. Gen. Psychiatry*, 27: 349-353, 1972.

15   Buglass, D., et al.: "A Scale for Predicting Subsequent Suicidal Behavior," *Brit. J. Psychiatry*, 124: 573-578, 1974.

16   Seiden, Richard: "The Problem of Suicide on College Campuses," *J. School Health*, 41 (5): 243-248, 1971.

17   Adams, R. L., et al.: "Risk Taking Among Suicide Attempters," *J. Abnormal Psychol.*, 82: 262-267, 1973.

18   Carter, Hugh, and Paul C. Glick: *Marriage and Divorce: A Social and Economic Study*, Harvard University Press, Cambridge, Mass., 1970.

19   Duvall, Evelyn Mills: *Family Development*, 4th ed., J. B. Lippincott Company, Philadelphia, 1971.

20   Glick, Ira D., and David R. Kessler: *Marital and Family Therapy*, Grune & Stratton, New York, 1974.

21   Glick, Paul C.: "First Marriage and Remarriages," *Am. Sociol. Rev.*, 14, 726-734, 1949.

22   Kimmel, Douglas C.: *Adulthood and Aging*. John Wiley & Sons, Inc., New York, 1974.

23* Thompson, Lida E., Michael H. Miller, and Helen F. Bigler: *Sociology-Nurses and Their Patients in a Modern Society*, C. V. Mosby Company, St. Louis, 1975.

24* Krantzler, Mel: *Creative Divorce: A New Opportunity for Personal Growth*, J. B. Lippincott Company, Philadelphia, 1973.

25* Despert, J. Louise: *Children of Divorce*. Doubleday & Company, Inc., Garden City, N.Y., 1953.

26* Women in Transition, Inc.: *Women in Transition — A Feminist Handbook on Separation and Divorce*, Charles Scribner's Sons, New York, 1975.

27* Starr, Bernard D., and Harris S. Goldstein: *Human Development and Behavior, Psychology in Nursing*, Springer Publishing Co., Inc., New York, 1975.

*Starred items are of particular interest.

CHAPTER 2

Activity and the Young Adult

VIGNETTE

As Kim and Nora Smith, a young married couple, are making out their health-assessment forms, the nurse asks them to describe their daily exercise activities in recent years as well as their current ones. In high school Nora played a great deal of girls' intramural volleyball, but when she graduated and took a job in the city, commuting took so much time that she had to restrict her physical activity to weekends. Now she is the mother of a toddler, at home all day: "Chasing my son is all the exercise I need!" Kim was very active physically when he was in college, bicycling to and from the university and playing basketball almost daily. Now, as a salesperson, he spends much of his day driving from town to town in his large district. Kim and Nora agree that they felt better when they had more physical activity but are too busy now to schedule regular exercise. When they have a free evening, they feel too tired for physical activity.

EXERCISE AND ACTIVITY

The need for activity and exercise is the same for the young adult as for the adolescent, but changes in life-style often decrease opportunities. The young adult man with a new job may become involved only in spectator sports, with the result that his physical fitness deteriorates, his endurance falls off, and he feels less and less

21

inclined for participation. A young father may feel "too big" to keep on playing with bachelor friends, and friends tend to disperse as some go away to college and others to jobs elsewhere. As a husband, he has new demands, social and domestic, on his weekend time. A young mother like Nora Smith may think she is *very* active; but the activity is not necessarily, by itself, the right kind. Young men and women often take the emotional feeling of tiredness as a sign that they are getting adequate exercise, but this is not necessarily the case.

The tone of our society today presents other threats to good health. We surround our young adults with labor-saving devices and tempt them to buy with the message: "This is what you *need* and *deserve*." But these devices may decrease activity and interfere significantly with the proper amount of exercise a person should be getting. Recent research has demonstrated that three out of four young persons are unable to pass tests designed to evaluate physical fitness for their age.[1] Young adult females, ages 20 to 29, had the lowest rating of all groups tested. Exercise physiologists define physical fitness as a state in which the person is able to complete all the tasks of daily living without fatigue or exhaustion with energy left over for leisure or evening activities.[2,3] Physically fit young adults, then, should not feel worn out like Kim and Nora Smith. The primary health care nurse should help them assess their level of physical fitness so that they may restore it, if necessary, to the level they enjoyed during adolescence and maintain it there.

PHYSICAL FITNESS

Body weight is often considered an indicator of physical fitness, yet experience often shows us young adults who are desirably thin yet tire easily after climbing a single flight of stairs. "I guess I've been smoking too much lately," such a person may say; but smoking is not, alone, a satisfactory explanation for the lack of fitness.

Maltz, Zeller, and Chandler have established some helpful criteria to assess the physical fitness of the young adult.

> The physically fit person has: (1) a slower heart rate during exercise; (2) a more rapid recovery rate; (3) a lower blood pressure before, during, and following exercise; (4) a lower oxygen intake; and (5) less lactic acid in the blood during exercise.[3]

The nurse can encourage young adults to assess their own physical fitness and should suggest some experiments which can be done easily at home without special equipment.

Clients may be told to select a stair in their home and to step up and down on it for 1 minute.

1   Step up with the left foot, then the right foot.
2   Step down with the left foot, then the right foot.
3   Repeat the lifts at a pace of 30 steps per minute for a person weighing between 100 and 160 pounds.
4   Between 160 and 220 pounds, the rate should be between 20 and 30 steps per minute.

The moment the test is finished, the client should sit down and count his pulse. If the pulse rate is more than 120, he is in poor physical fitness.

If the rate is less than 120, he should repeat the 1-minute exercise immediately. If the pulse rate is over 120, he is in fair physical fitness.

If the rate of the second exercise is less than 120, he should repeat the 1-minute exercise immediately for a third time. If the pulse rate is over 120, he is in good physical fitness. If it is under 120 he is in excellent physical fitness.

Young adults who are interested in a more detailed evaluation of their physical fitness should be referred to *The New Aerobics* by Kenneth H. Cooper, M.P.H. This book includes simple activities that can be useful in evaluating and then maintaining physical fitness in adults.

EXERCISE REQUIREMENTS
Exercise is essential for many reasons. First, exercise plays an important role in the regulation of one's appetite. Inactive young adults are more likely to overeat than moderately active young adults.[2] Exercise also helps release bottled-up, emotional tensions. Emotional fatigue from worry over money, losing a job, illness in the family, marital troubles, or boredom can be alleviated by the right kind of exercise. Exercise aids sleep, retards the aging process, and helps keep body muscles firm. The heart is also protected by exercise.[1, 2, 4]

Whatever advantages modern technology offers us, it also presents us with problems primitive men never faced. As hunter and hunted, primitive man had plenty of exercise and an enormous appetite and was in prime physical condition. Today we eat too much and exercise too little. The cardiovascular system suffers; the heart and blood vessels begin to degenerate. It is entirely possible, however, for the well young adult, with a little thought and encouragement, to adopt activities which will keep him literally young in heart despite the dangers of current life-styles.

The best exercise is physical activity that exercises the heart. The exercise must increase the heart rate, require deeper breathing, and encourage the blood vessels to expand and to carry more oxygen. Chasing a toddler may meet these requirements, of course, but only sporadically and briefly; and the key words in exercise are "regular" and "sustained." Young adults need to be encouraged to give more attention to calisthenics. Many young people enjoy participating in exercise programs offered on television, but while these types of exercise maintain muscle tone and strength, they do not in themselves provide sufficient exercise for the heart. A good combination might be calisthenics every other day, alternating with jogging, bicycling, or swimming.

It is to be remembered, however, that type and amount of exercise may vary considerably. Popular sports like bowling and golfing provide only minimal exercise for the heart. Bicycle riding, hiking, dancing, jogging, swimming, horseback riding, rope jumping, tennis, handball, badminton, hockey, rowing, skating, skiing, and volleyball all provide adequate exercise when done regularly. Again, exercise should be regular; weekend jogging is not the answer. Ideally, some exercise should be taken daily, though studies show no significant difference between daily exercise and exercise taken four times a week. The value of exercise cannot be stored; after a layoff of 3 weeks, the system reverts to a state comparable to that of no exercise at all.[1,2] For a four-times-a-week program, the person might consider jogging twice a week and swimming and hiking once; or jumping rope one day, bicycling to the store the next, and going on a hike and taking a horseback ride on the weekend.

Since habit formation is extremely important for the young adult, it is desirable to try to include a little strenuous exercise every day. With imagination, there is plenty of opportunity for a well young adult to do this. One young woman, for instance, does her laundry in the basement, and then, instead of taking the elevator back to her apartment, runs up the three flights of stairs; another woman parks her car in the far corner of the shopping center and runs to and from the stores she visits.

Exercise requirements vary for each individual. Women, particularly those who may be homebound, often can include beneficial activities in their daily schedule. See Table 2-1.

If the well young adult is aware of the importance of exercise to health, his or her ingenuity will be equal to the challenge of getting it.

While jogging, bicycling, and swimming are perhaps the best

TABLE 2-1[5]

Activity	Calories expanded per hour
Bedmaking	234
Desk work	132
Driving a car	168
Farm work in field	438
Handball	612
Horseback riding (trot)	480
Ironing (standing up)	252
Lawn mowing (hand mower)	462
Piano playing	150
Preparing a meal	198
Scrubbing of floors	216
Sitting and eating	84
Sitting and knitting	90
Sitting in a chair reading	72
Skiing (downhill)	594
Sleeping (basal metabolism)	60
Standing up	138
Sweeping	102
Swimming (leisurely)	300
Walking (2.5 miles per hour)	216
Walking downstairs	312

forms of exercise for the well young adult, each has some factors which need to be considered.

Bicycling has recently become very popular, and its appeal is increasing steadily in both urban and rural areas. A young adult should bicycle at a speed that elevates the pulse rate to between 135 and 160 beats per minute and then sustain that speed, if possible, for 20 minutes. With the increasing popularity of bicycling, however, there is increasing concern for the cyclist on roads heavily traveled by automobiles because of the high incidence of automobile-bicycle accidents. Also, for the urban rider, there may be danger in the amount of carbon monoxide inhaled, because bicycling encourages the rider to breathe more deeply.

In many parts of the country and for much of the year, swimming requires access to a pool. Swimming laps provides a good way to calculate the quality of the exercise. The swimmer should take his pulse after 5 minutes. If the pulse rate is between 135 and 160 beats per minute, he should continue swimming at the same speed for a total of 20 minutes.

Jogging, perhaps the most valuable of these exercises, has become very popular, but the nurse should be aware of several guidelines before recommending it. Before beginning to jog, any young adult over the age of 35 should have a complete physical examination, including a stress electrocardiogram (ECG). This is particularly important since he may already have silent heart disease. Others who should be checked by a physician before beginning a jogging program are those who smoke more than one pack of cigarettes a day or who have a close relative who suffered a heart attack before the age of 50. Still others are those who have hypertension and/or elevated triglycerides (serum cholesterol). Finally, no one more than 25 percent overweight should begin an exercise program without first consulting a doctor.

The process of jogging itself should be conducted with certain safeguards of which the nurse should be aware. Joggers should allow at least 5 minutes to warm up, since it is important to allow the cardiovascular system to cope gradually with an increase in exercise. Once a person's heart rate is up to 135 to 160 beats per minute, exercise should continue for 20 minutes. "Cooling down" is as important as warming up, and joggers should reduce their exercise slowly and never stop suddenly. After jogging, they should walk for a few minutes. The same caution to cool off gradually applies to swimming, tennis, bicycling, and all of the other strenuous exercises.

REST AND RELAXATION

The proper amount of rest and relaxation is as important to physical fitness in the young adult as the proper amount of activity, but it may be even harder for young adults to discipline themselves to secure it. This is perhaps the time above all others in life which offers new and challenging demands, and heavy pressures come with them. "I'm tired," says Kim, "but it won't kill me to sit up tonight and get that sales chart done." "The doctor said the baby's colic was under control," says Nora, "but I just can't get to sleep when I keep thinking I'll hear him cry." The nurse must be persuasive and convince them that sleep, and the right kind of sleep, is important and indispensable.

STAGES OF SLEEP

Sleep is not just sleep. Few people fall asleep instantaneously. The transition from the stage of waking to that of sleeping is marked by a series of physical changes which continue throughout the four stages into which sleep is divided. (See Figure 2-1.) The ritual of sleep begins as the individual moves from a state of waking in which the electroencephalogram (EEG) is pinched and irregular, to a state of relaxation. Respiration then becomes more regular, the pulse grows

Waking State
EEG: Brain waves pinched and irregular scrawl; rapid irregular brain charges—low voltage.

Two major classes of sleep:
REM (rapid eye movement) class of sleep—activated sleep state
non-REM (non-rapid eye movement) class of sleep is found in 4 stages

Relaxation
Respiration grows regular—pulse even, temperature declines, aimless thoughts.

Border of Waking/Sleeping
EEG: Scrawl not so pinched, bursts at an even rhythm 9-13 per second; alpha rhythm relaxed and serene, drifting of mind like raft on water.

Stage I Sleep
Light state of sleep; increase in moderate brain waves; voltage and frequency interspersed, and bursts resembling wire spindles; REM appears here in Stage I.

Alpha rhythm changes, eyes begin to roll slowly. Images or vague thoughts as one begins to traverse gates of consciousness. Sudden spasm, myoclonic jerk—may awaken one momentarily. Normal sign of movement to sleep—sleeper easily awakened.

Stage II Sleep
Enters this stage with images and fragmentary dreams; brain waves grow longer and slower, medium depth sleep.

Stage III Sleep
EEG: Large, slow waves 1 per second; may be reached about 20 minutes after falling asleep; brain waves slower but with increasing voltage.

Stage IV Sleep
EEG: Large slow waves at high voltage. Deep sleep follows Stage III in a few minutes; sinks into bottomless oblivion (lasting 10-20 minutes). Exceedingly hard to awaken (sleep of the weary); if awakened will be confused, remember nothing. When bedwetting, sleep walking, nightmares, or screams occur—restorative sleep.

REM (rapid eye movement) periods in sleep occur periodically throughout the sleep cycle at regular intervals of 85-110 minutes (average of every 90 minutes). This would equal approximately 4-5 episodes of dream activity (when breath and pulse become irregular, penile erections occur, but body feels flaccid; if awakened before muscle tone returns will feel paralyzed). Character of sleep changes throughout the night; as sleep becomes lighter by morning, REM episodes are longer, more bizarre. Each person, however, has his own REM pattern which changes throughout the life cycle.

REM sleep is not a unity but a conjunction of physiological rhythms and experiences essential to one's well-being.

Sleep needs change with the life cycle
REM normally decreases markedly from birth to the age of five years. Children and young people spend much more of the early portion of night in deep sleep (when growth hormones reach peak in the blood). Depth of sleep begins to vanish after age 30. Longer periods of lighter sleep in declining years. Extra REM during early years may be related to mental growth.

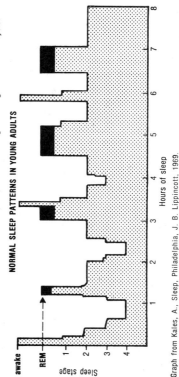

NORMAL SLEEP PATTERNS IN YOUNG ADULTS

Hours of sleep

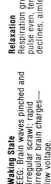

Sleep stage

awake
REM
1
2
3
4

Graph from Kales, A., Sleep, Philadelphia, J. B. Lippincott, 1969.

FIGURE 2-1 Sleep patterns and stages.

more even, and body temperature declines. At this stage, an individual may have fleeting, aimless thoughts. Next, the EEG becomes less pinched and achieves an even rhythm of from 9 to 13 cycles per second. The individual may feel as if he is "floating" into sleep. At this stage, the young adult may be awakened easily. Consciousness then begins to decrease, and the individual enters stage I sleep.

This is a light stage of sleep in which rapid eye movements (REM) can be observed. There is an increase in brain wave activity, perhaps due to the presence of REM or dream activity. During this period, breath and pulse become irregular and penile erections occur although the body feels flaccid. If an individual is awakened from REM sleep before muscle tone has returned, he may feel paralyzed. REM sleep occurs periodically throughout the night in 60-minute to 90-minute intervals with longer REM episodes as sleep becomes lighter toward the end of sleep.

Stage II is a medium-deep sleep that occurs when the brain waves grow longer and slower.

In stage III, the EEG waves slow to 1 per second, but there is increasing voltage. This stage may occur 20 minutes after falling asleep.

Stage IV, or deep sleep, quickly follows stage III. This stage can last from 10 to 20 minutes, and it is very hard to awaken someone during this period. Nightmares, screams, and restorative sleep occur during this stage. Stage IV decreases and is absent by the time light-sleep states are found in the morning in the adult.

The depth of sleep, marked by the length of stage IV, begins to decrease after age 30.[6] Thus, a normal night's sleep is not one continuous level plane but a series of repeated cycles in which at some intervals the individual returns to a near-waking state.

FUNCTIONS OF SLEEP

Much sleep research remains to be done, but the different types of sleep—dream sleep, sometimes called rapid eye movement (REM) sleep, and deep sleep—are well established. Each has a function that is indispensable to physical well-being.

For many years, deep sleep has been recognized as a necessary healer. Its function apparently is to counteract the effects of physical tiredness. It is restorative after fatigue, pain, or injury. "Tired Nature's sweet restorer, balmy sleep," said Edward Young in *Night Thoughts* more than 200 years ago. Anabolism and macromolecule synthesis occur in deep sleep. Jovanic (1971) observed that the mechanism of the restorative process is not clear, but it probably involves repair and growth of synaptic endings. Deep sleep repairs, reorganizes, and forms the new connections in the catecholaminergic neuronal systems which are required for focused attention, learning, and secondary process. During deep sleep, the macromolecules that are synthesized are used later in the dream periods in the process of restoring and building synaptic connections.[7]

One of the functions of REM sleep, it is thought, is restoration and the easing of psychic strain after anxiety and depression brought about by new learning situations. Jovanic suggests that

> psychologically it makes sense to think of this as connecting recent information with old pathways or "filing system." Insofar as we become conscious of this process in dreaming, it is manifested as the connection of "day residue" material with old emotional pathways such as wishes and fears.[7]

EEG tests show "reorganized pulses" cementing these new connections. The importance of REM sleep for the young adult confronted with new learning of all types is therefore apparent. Since it functions in reversing the tiredness occurring after new learning or other mental and emotional work—particularly to restore recently acquired ego functions, ability to focus attention, learning and memory mechanisms[7]—young adults, be they laboratory researchers, sales representatives, or young mothers, must provide for it or take the consequences of impairment of performance and behavior.

SLEEP REQUIREMENTS

Sleep is both individual and cyclical. There are no simple tools, such as those in the field of activity, by which the nurse can assess the sleep requirements of her clients. To a great extent the nurse must rely upon their observations while furnishing them with the latest scientific data and thus emphasizing the importance of the habit-forming decisions they must make for themselves.

The average number of hours young adults sleep is approximately 8 hours per day, though this varies significantly between individuals. Research is currently being conducted to determine the variables, both physical and psychological, which affect sleep requirements. The nurse needs to take advantage of the latest research on the types, stages, and functions of sleep.

SLEEP RESEARCH

Until now the importance of sleep and relaxation to the health of young adults has not received its merited attention in the areas of health maintenance and promotion, but much important research is now being conducted in this field.

In an experiment in which students were partially deprived of sleep for 8 weeks, sustained attention showed a marked decrease over a 30-minute period. There was also a reduction in rectal temperatures in stage IV sleep and a reduction in the alpha density throughout the experimental period. Although the implications of these significant physiological changes are yet to be researched, the decrease in efficiency is evident.

Other studies have been done on the implications of working evening and night shifts.[8] The quality of day sleep after night work, it was found, differs from normal night sleep in that there is a significant shortening of the sleep cycle. As a consequence, the worker may expect more "tiredness" than he felt when working on day shifts, even though he may think he is receiving the same amount of sleep.

Young adults who deprive themselves of sleep for days at a time, for whatever reason, may experience changes in personality and performance. Hallucinations and psychosis can occur, and following 48 hours of sleep deprivation, severe behavioral changes, such as suspiciousness, depression, aggression, and withdrawal, may also occur.

Under competitive modern pressures, students are tempted to cut down on sleep to add hours to their study day. Similarly, men and women anxious to make a success of a new job will bring home night work in order to impress the boss. But this behavior is based on a fallacy. Sleep is not an expendable asset. Studies indicate that the brain catecholamines, especially norepinephrine, take part in higher central-nervous system functions such as alertness, learning, and memory. Because REM sleep restores balance to the catecholamines and functional integrity to the neuronal system, and deep sleep also repairs and is involved in the synaptic endings of the neurons, the day's learning is connected and filed with other pathways.[7] The nurse must show the student, the office worker, and the young mother, that sleep relates to learning, and nothing can replace it. To skimp on sleep is to risk impaired learning and physiological damage.

When an individual tries to recover lost sleep by sleeping longer hours, most of the time will be spent in REM sleep but it does not make up for the lost REM sleep. Similarly, reducing sleep time does not yield a "miniature" of a full night's sleep. The person remains mostly in stage IV and has very little of the REM sleep needed to carry out various roles and responsibilities optimally.

INSOMNIA

Perhaps every nurse has heard the young adult's common complaint about insomnia. It may result from stress, anxiety, lack of exercise, or any combination of these. There are three types of insomnia: *initial*, or the inability to fall asleep; *intermittent*, or frequent waking during the night; and *terminal*, early waking with inability to go back to sleep. The first is the most common and may attack those in whom the need for sleep is very great, particularly after a day of much new learning or emotional stress, anxiety, or depression.

The exact mechanism of "falling asleep" is not yet completely understood. We are all familiar with the feeling of drowsiness that occurs after heavy meals and with the homespun prescription of a glass of warm milk at bedtime. One study on the effects of L-tryptophase on sleep shows that this enzyme is indeed helpful, as are foods containing it, such as cottage cheese, meat, or nuts.[7]

Many young adults, unfortunately, are not satisfied with so simple a technique and therefore resort to medication, of which many types are available without prescription. Since this may lead to psychological addiction, the nurse would do well to discuss with her clients the possibility of treating insomnia through changes in life-style or diet. Sedatives significantly reduce REM sleep; and when the drug is withdrawn, REM sleep continues to be reduced, causing insomnia, nightmares, fatigue, and sensitivity to pain. These symptoms can persist for 5 weeks. Medication should be prescribed only when other primary interventions have failed.

Some simple information may be helpful to insomniacs. Many people do not know that in the normal sleep cycle the sleeper goes through the four stages of sleep a number of times every night. With every return to stage I sleep, the sleeper is very close to being in the wakeful state. The average cycle is 90-plus minutes. If a sleeper wakes frequently, he might check to see if he is starting a new cycle. Knowing that the levels of consciousness normally change frequently during the night may relieve his anxiety when he wakes up at 1:30 a.m. (Contrary to popular belief, sleep becomes lighter, not heavier, as the night progresses.) A simple change might help him establish a rhythm to harmonize with the rhythms of sleep. Tossing and turning all night will achieve nothing more for him than a tired feeling the next day; but he might try a nap after dinner and then a wakeful period of an hour or so in the night, which, free from anxiety, he could utilize to good advantage. Quiet music, a dim light, or counting sheep, on the other hand, may all contribute to a state of monotony or boredom in which the cerebral cortex does not respond to the reticular formation.

The role of the nurse is to provide anticipatory guidance of this nature, and she should also emphasize that sleep rhythms are an individual matter.

BASIC REST-ACTIVITY CYCLE
Waking as well as sleep is normally marked for adults by a 90-minute basic rest-activity cycle that is apparently related to gastric

contractions.[9] Human processes are rhythmical; indeed much of what we do and experience may be rhythmical. Health may be considered a matter of harmonious circadian rhythms (that is, rhythms of every 24-hour period). Altering body rhythms may be a serious matter which may eventually lead to illness. "The malaise, anorexia, and insomnia of the nurse who changes from day to night shift may be an example of a lack of integration of rhythmical phase relationships."[10] Luce suggests that ulcers and other symptoms appearing among workers on rotating shifts may indicate that stress and a desynchronization of circadian rhythms may lead to illness. Increasingly, we hear of the exhaustion and malaise of jet lag; it may be traceable to excessive internal desynchronization.[11]

For normal adults, there are 15 to 16 basic rest-activity cycles in each 24 hours; 5 of them usually occur in sleep, the remaining 10 or 11 in wakefulness. The resurgence of activity every 85 to 95 minutes probably represents a primitive hunger drive, accentuated by periodic gastric contractions. There is evidence that the mechanism is neurohormonal in character and depends upon the action of accumulated neurohormones on the central nervous system, specifically on the pontile reticular formation.[7]

Thus, as the primary health care nurse assesses the activity of the young adult, she needs to consider exercise, sleep, and waking activities. The young adult's work and leisure schedule represents his basic rest-activity schedule; accordingly, this schedule greatly influences other primary health care areas such as eating, drinking, and smoking. (See Chapter 3, Nutrition and the young adult.) How leisure time is spent is not only important now, but it is undoubtedly going to raise more and more problems as the workweek shortens and the amount of leisure time increases.

Since the young adult, as we know, is in a period of life that presents changes, the nurse should assess the normal day and then counsel as to necessary adaptations. (Refer to Chapter 1, on the changes in the young adult beginning on page 4.)

HAZARDS OF YOUNG ADULT ACTIVITY

Traveling is a frequent activity of the young adult. Most often this involves the automobile or other motor vehicles. In 1974, over 25,000 deaths occurred in the 25- to 44-year-old age group from motor vehicle accidents alone.[12] Death by motor accident is as common and as taken for granted as was the heavy infant mortality of the Middle Ages. Highways are made safer, driver education is provided, and cars are equipped with one safety device after another, yet the rate of accidents climbs steadily. Research is needed, for we do not know the interrelationships between behavior and reaction on the one hand, and psychological and physiological stress on the other, or how either affects driving performance.

There are various reliable predictive factors the nurse can offer. One is the use of seat belts. The accident potential increases in inverse proportion to the percentage of time that drivers and passengers use seat belts; the more often you fasten your seat belt, the less likely you are to have an accident. Conversely, the accident factor increases in direct proportion to the number of miles driven. If driver A drives his car 10 times as many miles in a year as driver B, his chance of accident is 10 times greater.[13] Though it almost seems that young adults believe freedom to drive a car is one of the freedoms promised by the Founding Fathers, the nurse might at least suggest that a traveling salesperson whose car is on the road 5 days a week should look around for activities in his neighborhood for the weekend instead of taking the car out for another 500 miles.

Combining medication and driving is dangerous. We need more research to provide information about the effects of drugs on drivers, but it is already known that some drugs (such as antidepressants, analgesics, anticonvulsants, and muscle relaxants) impair driving performance. Even some antibiotics, like streptomycin, can produce dizziness and loss of balance. Of great importance is the synergistic relationship between these commonly prescribed drugs and that other drug, alcohol. Even one drink at lunch can have an explosive effect when added to medication.[14] Young adults who take routine medications need to be very conscious of the dangers they may be incurring when they drive.

The effect of lack of sleep on the incidence of accidents also requires more investigation. In one study 28 young male adults were deprived of sleep and then given periodic tests for reaction times, discrimination reactions, reading, concentration, and attention. The results offer evidence for a correlation between lack of sleep and propensity for having an accident. Even after relatively short periods of sleep deprivation, "perception, concentration, attention and adaptability with respect to new or rapidly changing situations were so impaired that, at critical moments, rapid and sensible reactions were no longer guaranteed."[7] A significant and disquieting factor in this study was that the subjects assessed their own performance as better than it actually was. The nurse whose client is a truck driver or salesperson who is tempted to do, indeed rewarded for, long-distance driving without adequate stops for rest, exercise, and sleep would do well to emphasize this information. But any young adults about to take a trip should be made aware of the risks they run if they neglect proper rest.

The most significant factor in accident potential is the individual's drinking habits. Alcoholics, defined by insurance actuarials as those who take 41 or more drinks a week, represent 4 percent of the population and cause 50 percent of the number of fatal accidents.[6] (Alcoholism will be discussed in detail in Chapter 8.) Heavy social, definite excess (25 to 40 drinks per week) and mild social excess (7 to 24 drinks per week) represent risks proportionately serious.[13] In discussing drinking habits, the nurse should not forget to inform the young adult of how drinking raises his car accident potential.

Another area that needs further investigation is that of suicide and its relation to motor vehicle accidents. Many so-called accidents are believed to be suicides. A client's emotional health then may be a significant factor in evaluating the risks for accidents.

A few rules might help young adults to avoid car accidents:

1   Keep your car in good working condition, check your brakes, and see that your tires grip the road.
2   Use your seat belts especially on short trips.
3   Watch the road, not the scenery or your passengers.
4   Don't let pets or children loose in the car.
5   On a long trip, stop for a rest break about every 100 miles and don't drive over 6 hours a day.
6   Don't drive if you have taken medication, are upset or angry, or have something on your mind more pressing than driving.
7   And above all: If you drink, don't drive; if you drive, don't drink.

There are, of course, other accident possibilities for the young adult, notably motorcycles, firearms, and drowning. Statistically speaking, however, they are relatively unimportant when compared to automobile accidents.

OCCUPATIONAL HAZARDS

Many young adults are not aware of the potential for injury or death involved in different types of occupations. We now have statistical data available which will help the primary health care nurse counsel young adult clients in this area. Because the young adult years are often a time of searching for life-long lines of work, the nurse may very well play a significant role not only in offering advice about what to expect in a current job, but in what to look for in selecting an occupation. The following list represents the ten most dangerous occupations:[12]

1   Fire fighting
2   Mining
3   Police work
4   Lumber
5   Quarry
6   Construction
7   Mining, surface
8   Cement
9   Foundary
10   Clay and mineral products

Clearly, this information suggests guidelines for the choice of occupation.

However, every nurse should also be aware that 90 percent of accidents are caused by human failure, be it poor mental health, alcoholism, stress, or attitudes. "When a client reveals an unconcern or a feeling that accidents are uncontrollable, the nurse must make some attempt to offer guidance in terms of changing his attitudes."[15]

The nurse also needs to be aware of the Occupational Safety and Health Act, particularly as it relates to the health and safety needs of workers. Many companies have fewer than 500 employees and because of this, many clients may not have access to an occupational health nurse. Hence the primary health care nurse may be the most appropriate person for assessing the hazards of the work environment and serving the health and safety needs of workers.

BIBLIOGRAPHY
1   Bailey, D. A., R. J. Shapard, R. L. Mirwald, and G. A. McBride: "A Current View of Canadian Cardiorespiratory Fitness," *Canadian Med. Assoc. J.*, III: 25-30, 1974.
2*   Cooper, Kenneth H.: *The New Aerobics*, Bantam Books, Inc., New York, 1970.
3   Maltz, Stephan, Verne Zellmer, and Harold Chandler: *College Health Science*, W. C. Brown Company Publishers, Dubuque, Iowa, 1973.
4   Germain, C. P.: "Exercise Makes the Heart Grow Stronger," *Am. J. Nursing*, 71 (6) 2169-2173, 1972.
5   *Nutrition Almanac*, Nutrition Search, Inc., McGraw-Hill Book Company, New York, 1975.
6   Sutterly, Doris Cook, and Gloria Ferraro Donnelly: *Perspectives in Human Development: Nursing Throughout The Life Cycle*, J. B. Lippincott Company, Philadelphia, 1973.
7*   Jovanic, U. J., ed.: *The Nature of Sleep*, Gustav Fischer Verlag, Stuttgart, Germany, 1971.
8   Felton, Geraldene: "Body Rhythm Effects on Rotating Work Shifts," *Nursing Digest*, 4: 29-32, 1976.

9   Kleitman, Nathaniel: *Sleep and Wakefulness*, rev. ed., The University of Chicago Press, Chicago, 1963.

10   German, M. Leah: "Conscious Repatterning of Human Behavior," *Am. J. Nursing*, 76: 1752–1754, 1975.

11   Luce, G. G.: *Biological Rhythms in Psychiatry and Medicine*, Dover Publications, Inc., New York, 1970.

12   National Safety Council (Statistics Division), *Accident Facts* J. L. Recht, director, Chicago, 1975.

13   Robbins, Lewis C., and Jack H. Hall: *How to Practice Prospective Medicine*, Methodist Hospital of Indiana, Indianapolis, 1970.

14* "Drugs and Alcohol," *Am. J. Nursing*, 76: 65, 1976.

15   Brown, Mary Louise: "The Quality of the Work Environment," *Am. J. Nursing*, 75: 1755–1760, 1975.

16* "Effects of Hypnotics on Sleep Patterns, Dreaming, and Mood State: Laboratory and Home Subjects," *Biological Psychiatry*, 1: 235–241, 1969.

17* Kales, A., ed.: *Sleep: Physiology and Pathology*, J. B Lippincott Company, Philadelphia, 1969.

18* Petre-Quadens, Olga, and John Schlag, ed.: *Basic Sleep Mechanism*, Academic Press, Inc., New York, 1974.

19* Cooper, Mildred, and Kenneth H. Cooper, *Aerobics for Women*, Bantam Books, Inc., New York, 1972.

*Starred items are of particular interest.

CHAPTER 3

Nutrition and the Young Adult

Young adulthood is a time when the individual begins to establish his adult eating habits. Frequently the young adult is very interested in foods and may be more amenable to dietary counseling than he will be at any other time in his life. It is also a time of food fads and diet experimentation.

DIETARY ASSESSMENT

The first step in dietary counseling is for the primary health care nurse to do a thorough dietary assessment. This assessment should include a comparision of the actual caloric intake with the normal caloric requirements established for this individual. Caloric requirements require consideration of climate, occupation, amount of physical activity, mental effort, emotional state, age, body size, and individual metabolism; and while charts may be helpful, the nurse must always adjust these figures for each individual[1-4] by calculating how much energy is expended each day. This assessment should also include the basic nutrients, vitamins, and minerals, as well as the basic food groups. (Refer to Dietary Assessment, Chap. 16.)

THE YOUNG ADULT DIET

The dietary needs of the young adult are not the same as those of the adolescent. Both males and females need less calcium and protein than they did as adolescents.[5] Males need more vitamins C, E, and B, and more riboflavin, but less niacin, thiamine, calcium, phosphorus, iodine, magnesium, and vitamin A. Females need more vitamin C, but less niacin, thiamine, calcium, phosphorus, iodine, and magnesium.[1,2,4]

Young adult males should include a glass of orange juice (vitamin C) in their diet every day, should substitute whole wheat for white bread (vitamins B_6 and B_{12}), use vegetable oils (vitamin E) and eat plenty of leafy vegetables (also vitamin E) and fish and cheese (vitamin B_{12}).

Young adult females should be particularly careful to include foods that contain vitamin C: citrus fruits, strawberries, cantaloupe, tomatoes, green peppers, and broccoli. Since many young women are anemic, particularly during menstruation, they should regularly include in their diet food high in iron: organ meats (liver, kidney, etc.), eggs, fish, poultry, blackstrap molasses, leafy vegetables, and dried fruits. Some physicians may even prescribe iron supplements for women, since it is often difficult to secure enough iron in the diet.

One of the most disturbing features of modern American nutrition is iron deficiency in the diet of many women. There is a real sex difference in the need for iron which is often ignored. From age 12 to 18, the male needs 18 milligrams of iron daily, but after the age of 18, he needs only 10 milligrams of iron. In contrast, females need 18 milligrams of iron from age 10 to 55. Often, a woman may eat the same diet as a man, thereby receiving 10 milligrams of iron. It is adequate for him, but meets only half the requirement for her. Approximately one-third of all American women between the ages of 10 and 55 are anemic (define anemic as being iron-deprived) and receive only one-third of their daily requirement of iron.[2] The symptoms of anemia are mild and may include fatigue, shortness of breath, and depression. A woman may have no idea that they are related to her diet.

Young adults should also be counseled to use only iodized salt and at the same time to salt food sparingly. In the inland parts of the country, away from the oceans, goiter may develop due to lack of iodine in the diet. Iodized salt will prevent this. However, large amounts of salt in any diet are unwise, since salt can contribute to hypertension. Because many foods, particularly processed foods, contain salt, it is a good practice either to salt food while cooking and to put no salt shaker on the table, or—perhaps preferable since salt sometimes destroys vitamins during cooking—to keep no salt shaker by the stove but to add salt at the table. Herbs and spices such as oregano, parsley, and cinnamon are a flavorable substitute for salt.

Today most young adults are familiar with the four basic food groups, but they may not know how many servings of each group they need. It may help if a list of the four basic food groups could be hung on the wall in a prominent place, perhaps over the kitchen sink or next to the kitchen table. It may also help for the nurse to encourage her clients to assess their own diets and eating habits. Frequently young adults will comment that they "don't eat right" or "don't eat a lot of things that they should." Often their diets may be reasonably well balanced, or deficient in only one or two foods which could be easily added. People of this age often feel they should lose weight, and in doing so they eliminate an entire food group, such as bread, flour, and cereals, because they think it is fattening. Actually, whole grain bread is a valuable food; it provides many important vitamins and nutrients and offers a very efficient use of calories. No basic group should be eliminated.

DIET MODIFICATIONS

There is one food which all nutritionists agree could be reduced not only safely, but advantageously; sugar. Sugar is high in calories, and it contributes nothing to the diet but calories. The average American eats 105 pounds of cane and beet sugar and 15 pounds of corn syrup yearly, and those figures are rising constantly.[5] Honey and maple sugar contain some trace elements lacking in beet or cane sugar, but for all intents and purposes all these substances contribute only empty calories. (An exception among sweeteners is blackstrap molasses, which is rich in iron.) Furthermore, the relation of sugar to tooth decay is well established, and recent research is beginning to link sugar consumption with heart diseases.[6] Many young adults, particularly those who buy only 5 pounds of sugar a year or who don't like "sweet things," have difficulty believing they consume 105 pounds of sugar a year. The reason is that many prepared foods ranging from salad dressing and peanut butter to canned chicken soup contain hidden sugar. With so much hidden sugar, the young adult might want to modify the diet to cut down on such obvious sources of sugar as sweet rolls, jams, and candies.

In addition to the subject of sugar, a controversial question currently receiving a good deal of attention is: Should foods high in cholesterol and saturated fats be limited in the diet of a young adult? The American Heart Association recommends that adult consumption of eggs be limited to three a week and that foods high in saturated fats be replaced by those containing polyunsaturated fats (butter by margarine, beef by chicken). The relationship of increased cholesterol in the blood and the development of heart disease is as yet inconclusive. However, emerging evidence suggests that damage to arteries from a buildup of cholesterol in the bloodstream occurs much earlier than was previously supposed. As early as age 15 males should limit their consumption of eggs and foods high in saturated fats unless they know, by frequent testing, that their triglycerides and serum cholesterol are low.[5]

It has been determined statistically that adults with a high serum cholesterol and high triglycerides have 3 to 4 times as much risk of developing coronary heart disease as persons with a low serum cholesterol or triglycerides.[5] Since these amounts can easily be determined by laboratory tests, the nurse should encourage her young adult clients to have such testing done as a part of the annual physical. If the tests show a slow rise in the levels of cholesterol in the blood, the diet can be modified. Those young adults who by heredity carry a risk factor for heart disease should modify their diet, particularly if they also have elevated serum cholesterol or triglycerides.

The ongoing question as to whether or not eggs contribute significantly to increased cholesterol in the bloodstream has been intensified by research which indicates that eggs, although undoubtedly high in cholesterol, also contain high amounts of choline, a substance that acts as an emulsifier in the circulatory system and therefore may prevent the buildup of cholesterol.[7] Eggs are a valuable and economical food source for protein, especially for pregnant women.

The following lists contain foods both high and low in cholesterol and saturated fats:

Food High in Cholesterol and Saturated Fats:

Eggs	Frankfurters
Beef	Whole milk
Sausage, cold cuts	Sour cream
Organ meats	Butter
Goose	Solid shortening
Lamb, pork	Commercial bakery goods

Foods Low in Cholesterol and Saturated Fats:

Poultry (except duck, goose)	Low-fat cheeses (cottage cheese)
Fish	Skim milk ice cream
Fruits	Margarine
Vegetables	Liquid cooking oil
Whole grain products	

Some young adults look upon butter as a status symbol, but they should be encouraged to use margarine, even if they can afford the "real thing." Margarine is dietetically superior since it is lower in cholesterol and saturated fat. Salad oils and margarines that are high in polyunsaturates include safflower oil, sunflower oil, and corn oil. On a margarine label the identification of the oil should come first, followed by the identification of the hydrogenated oil. The process of hydrogenation, which makes the margarine firm, also increases the amount of saturated fats in the margarine. Therefore, clients should be encouraged to use the softer margarine, as it contains less hydrogenated oil and less saturated fat. The first ingredient listed on the label of highly polyunsaturated margarine should be *liquid* corn, sunflower, or safflower oil.

Another controversial question currently under discussion is the presence of additives in our diet. Our food supply currently contains some additives that act as preservatives, and most experts agree that, so far, they seem to be useful.[5,7] However, our food also contains other additives that act as food colorings, flavorings, taste enhancers, and stabilizers. For these there is less justification, particularly when, as now seems to be true, they can be harmful. Potassium and sodium nitrates and nitrites have been used as food preservatives for years, but recent research now suggests that they might be carcinogenic.[8] Magee suggests that

> Nitrates are not potentially harmful unless they are converted into nitrites. Nitrates may be found naturally in water, and they are present in high concentration in such vegetables as beets, spinach, carrots and cabbage. However, nitrites are added to more than 12 billion pounds of food each year in the U.S. The highest concentrations of nitrites are found in hotdogs, bacon, ham, lunch meats, smoked fish, and some imported cheeses. When foods are spot checked, considerably more nitrates have been found repeatedly. Large amounts of nitrites are considered potentially dangerous because nitrites can react with amines in the human stomach to form nitrosamines.[9]

We do not know whether nitrosamines can cause cancer in man, though we do know that nitrosamines have induced malignant tumors in a wide range of laboratory animals. In addition to being formed by nitrites, nitrosamines are also formed from secondary amines and quaternary ammonium compounds found in foods and drugs. Major sources of amines include decongestant medications, cigarette smoking, beer, and ingested pesticides. Among the other drugs known to form carcinogenic nitrosamines by interaction with nitrites are oxytetracycline (Terramycin and others), aminopyrine, disulfiram (Antabuse), nikethamide (Coramine), tolazamide (Tolinase). Nitrosamines themselves have also been found in food, especially in bacon after frying.[10]

On the positive side, nitrates and nitrites are effective preservatives. Their main value is in the prevention of the growth of *Clostridium botulinum* in meats and fish.[11,12] There are other ways in which these foods may be preserved, but we need more time to evaluate the effectiveness, safety, and economic feasibility of these methods.[13,14] While research has not yet reached the stage of giving us a definite answer about such additives, the primary health care nurse should inform her clients of the possibility that they may be dangerous. This is particularly important for those who have a family history of cancer. These clients should be advised to avoid foods high in additives, particularly the nitrates and nitrites. They could, for instance, replace bacon or sausage with freshly cooked meats, or select those containing no preservatives for occasional use.

Another additive now receiving some attention as possibly being carcinogenic is Red Dye number 2. This additive is used for coloring in a wide variety of foods such as gelatin, lunch meats, and hot dogs. Since this additive contributes no preserving qualities, but is only used to make the color more pleasing, clients might be counseled to play it safe and to avoid foods with this type of additive.

DIET AND PSYCHOSOCIAL FACTORS

For both men and women, young adulthood is often a time to assume responsibility for preparing their own food, sometimes individually and sometimes in groups. The primary health care nurse will want to find out how much her clients know about cooking. Can they prepare food so that vital nutrients are not lost? Do they know that vegetables which are soaked in water lose many of their water-soluble vitamins? Are they aware that water in which vegetables have been cooked should be saved for soups or vegetable cocktails, since it contains valuable nutrients not to be wasted on the kitchen sink? There are many excellent books and pamphlets to help young adults in the area of nutrition and food preparation. (Refer to starred items in the bibliography at the end of this chapter.)

Young married people often begin their married life by overeating. In some families it is considered a good sign if the husband puts on weight since it shows that his wife is "taking good care of him." The new wife may find it hard to cook for only two if she has been in the habit of cooking at home for parents and siblings. If both the husband and wife are working, they may have money to spend on delicacies which they formerly could not afford. On the other hand, working may leave very little time to prepare foods, and may lead to heavy dependence on convenience foods and TV dinners, which are often high in calories and low in nutrients. Eating out in restaurants, which is especially common for single young adults, can also contribute to poor nutritional habits and overeating.

In addition, the young couple may not take the time to eat breakfast, may either skip lunch or overeat at lunch, and will then eat a huge evening meal. Because the body needs nutrients throughout the day, eating one or two huge meals a day is a poor nutritional practice. Because night eating or eating one huge meal a day produces more insulin, which in turn makes the body's metabolism of these calories into fat more efficient, these practices can contribute to overeating and obesity. (The problems of weight reduction and obesity will be covered in Part II, The Middle Adult, because the problems are often most acute during middle age.)

Socializing for the young adult, whether it is entertaining in his own home or attending a party, is frequently accompanied with food. This may be high caloric, empty-calorie snack foods or special delicacies prepared by the host or hostess for the occasion.

The nurse should assess how much the young adult relies on convenience foods. She also needs to be sensitive to whether money for food is a problem. All of these psychosocial factors should be considered by the nurse doing a thorough nutritional assessment, so that she can provide the client with anticipatory guidance. The nurse needs to be prepared to answer the nutritional questions of the young adult or know where to go for the answers. Some young adults may add massive doses of vitamins and minerals to their diets. Others may diet by drinking water and having only a vitamin pill for breakfast because they think that vitamins are an acceptable food substitute, which they are not. Since it is impossible to include material on all of the practices related to vitamin and mineral supplements, the nurse should use the resources she has available in her community or hospital as well as the books and pamphlets listed at the end of this chapter to answer questions in this area.

ALTERNATE DIETS

For some people, nutrition is simply a matter of meeting health needs; they eat to live. But for others, such as those interested in macrobiotics, it may be much more. For these individuals, eating is a matter not merely of physical needs, but also emotional and spiritual ones. Shimoda writes:

> Defined very simplistically, macrobiotics is a Far Eastern philosophy based on the yin-yang principle. The diet followed as part of this philosophy

has ten stages. At the lowest levels it consists of a variety of foods and is fairly well balanced. As progressive stages of the diet are reached however, various categories of foods are eliminated. The final diet consists of 100 percent cereals. Thus a person might be subsisting on brown rice and tea. If followed for a long time, such a diet is self-destructive.[15]

Register observes that in Zen macrobiotic diets

individuals who persist in following the more rigid diets are in great danger of developing serious nutritional deficiencies. Cases of scurvy, anemia, hypoproteinemia, hypocalcemia, emaciation due to starvation and other forms of malnutrition in addition to loss of kidney function due to restricted fluid intake have been reported, some of which have resulted in death.[16]

Many young adults are interested in eating more natural or organically grown foods and in discarding foods with preservatives or a high degree of processing. Many are becoming vegetarians, devoting themselves to the practice of eating lower on the food chain; that is, eating grain foods as they come from the fields rather than waiting to eat them in the form of meat into which they are processed by animals. Lappe suggests that such a diet may well be superior in quality to the ordinary diet.[17] Unfortunately, an uninformed nurse may respond automatically to a client's statements that he is practicing a vetegarian diet by suggesting that such a diet is inherently deficient or bad for him.

The nurse should know that a vegetarian diet is not necessarily the same thing as a Zen macrobiotic diet. Most nutritionists agree that vegetarian diets can be *entirely adequate w*ith careful planning to insure that all necessary nutrients are included.[17, 18, 4] It will take the nurse some time to work out with a vegetarian client everything he will need to include in his diet to receive all the necessary nutrients. Calcium, iron, riboflavin, and vitamin B, for instance, are all essential nutrients,[12] and they are found only marginally in all-plant diets.[18] On the other hand, some vegetarian diets often combine amino acids in such a way as to produce better-quality proteins than occur in the individual foods making up the combination. Thus these diets are not only adequate, but superior in quality.

There are three types of vegetarians. Some avoid only red meat and eat poultry and fish. Lacto-ovo-vegetarians avoid flesh food, but consume milk, cheese, and eggs. Finally, strict or pure vegans avoid all foods of animal origin. Obviously, planning for good nutrition becomes harder the more the choice of food is restricted; but an adequate diet is possible under any of these categories if the user is well informed. If any of these alternate diets is practiced by the client, the nurse must first accept it. She must then assess the adequacy of the diet with the client. If the nurse feels inadequate in her own food knowledge of vegetarian diets, she should consult many of the fine resources available to her.

Many young adults follow vegetarian diets, not for philosophical or spiritual reasons, but because they believe the practice is healthful. There is some data to support this view. Vegetarians usually have lower blood cholesterol levels than do meat eaters, partly due to the fact that they eat less fat and consume less cholesterol. One remarkable statistic is that the incidence of heart disease among Seventh Day Adventist males (vegetarians) is 40 percent lower than that of the average male population in California. Vegetarians also consume more fiber and roughage, and controlled studies testify that the feeding of legumes, which are high in fiber, has lowered the blood pressure of individuals studied. It is also reported that vegetarians experience a decreased incidence of cancer.[19] A current question not yet resolved is whether the higher incidence of cancer of the colon in industrialized countries is related to high fat intake (as in meat) or to low fiber intake.

DIET AND PREGNANCY

Pregnancy requires changes in diet and the period prior to pregnancy is of particular importance. The primary health care nurse plays a vital role in providing anticipatory guidance to the young adult female. Any woman who is planning on conceiving should be sure that she is not anemic and that her nutritional status is good. Often women are 2 or 3 months pregnant before their pregancy is confirmed and blood tests done to determine if the woman is anemic. This early period in which crucial developmental changes are occurring requires optimal nutritional status in the matter.

There are two common myths about maternal nutrition. One is that the fetus will get everything that it needs from the mother regardless of what she eats. The other is that the mother will instinctively crave and consume whatever the fetus needs. Both are false. Only nutrients in the mother's diet are available to the child. Therefore, the mother cannot afford to eat "junk" foods.[20]

The critical relationship that exists between the diet of the mother and the health of the fetus is not as widely recognized in the United States as it could be.

The United States ranks thirteenth among the nations of the world in infant mortality rates despite its position of wealth, medical knowledge, and skill. It ranks even lower (seventeenth) in the statistic of low birth weight babies. These infants have a much higher death rate and incidence of defects than do well-grown infants.[20]

It ought to be made clear to expectant mothers that during pregnancy the demands are enormous for nutrients to build tissues in the fetus, and for sources of energy. If these are not met, both mother and child will suffer.

In the fetus nutritional deficiencies will increase the incidences of congenital malformations, low birth weight babies, and perinatal death. In the mother, nutritional practices may produce or contribute to anemia, edema, and gastrointestinal disturbances. Inadequate nutrition will lower the ability of the pregnant woman to meet unusual stresses during or after pregnancy.[20]

VIGNETTE

Altoria is 21 years old and she is in her second trimester of pregnancy. She has a very low hemoglobin and is anemic. In discussing her diet with the nurse, she confides that she has an incredible craving for laundry starch. Some days she eats two boxes. She relates that her mother experienced the same phenomena all through her pregnancies. In further assessing Altoria's diet, the nurse discovers that she is also a pure vegan and does not eat any foods of animal origin, such as milk, cheese, eggs, or poultry. She and her husband are both students and are living on small incomes, so there is limited money to purchase food. She is interested in improving her diet because she understands the implications of anemia during pregnancy. She asks the nurse what diet modifications she should make.

Some women during pregnancy experience *pica*, the craving for strange foods or for nonfood substances, such as laundry starch, clay, frost from the freezer, and dirt. The nurse should be particularly conscientious in finding out whether or not a woman is experiencing pica. The problem with pica is usually not what is eaten but what is not eaten. Women who fill up on such things as starch have no room left for the foods they need and may experience severe nutritional deficiencies.

During her pregnancy, the mother should increase her caloric intake and meet a special demand for protein, calcium, iron, and vitamins A, B, C, and D (folic acid). [7, 21-23] A mother's average weight gain should be between 20 and 30 pounds, usually 25. Weight reduction should never be undertaken during pregnancy. It may be harmful both to the fetus and the mother, since it is usually accompanied by reduction in vitally needed nutrients essential to the growth process of the pregnancy. Women who suffer from edema sometimes restrict their salt intake; but salt-free diets are potentially dangerous during pregnancy, as is the use of diuretics. Studies indicate the need for sodium at this time.[24] A woman with edema

TABLE 3-1

| Nutrient | Amount | | Food sources |
	Non-pregnant	Pregnant	
Protein	46 g	76–100	Milk, cheese, eggs, meat, grains, legumes, and nuts
Calcium	800 mg	1200 mg	Milk, cheese, whole grains, leafy vegetables, egg yolk
Iron	18 mg	48–78 mg	Liver, meat, eggs, whole or enriched grains, leafy vegetables, nuts, legumes, dried fruits
Vitamins: A	4000 I.U.	5000 I.U.	Butter, cream, fortified margarine, green and yellow vegetables
B Complex	—	Increased	Meat, eggs, dairy products, grains, leafy vegetables
Folic acid	400 ug	800 ug	Liver, leafy vegetables
C	45 mg	60 mg	Citrus fruits, berries, melons, tomatoes, broccoli, chili peppers
D	0	400 I.U.	Fortified milk, fortified margarine
Calories	2100	2400	Carbohydrates, proteins, fats

should consult her physician and never prescribe medications for herself.

The nurse should be familiar with the normal changes in diet to provide the nutrients needed in pregnancy.[7,20,22] Table 3-1 may be helpful.

DIET MODIFICATIONS DURING PREGNANCY

During pregnancy it is important for the nurse to be supportive of the client-doctor relationship and to work closely in explaining diet modification. However, the primary health care nurse frequently helps her client to lessen some common complaints of pregnancy by suggesting some diet modifications. Nausea and vomiting, commonly called "morning sickness," is usually mild and limited to the first trimester. The nurse may advise her client to try the following to alleviate her nausea and vomiting:

1   Eat frequent small meals consisting chiefly of easily digested energy foods such as carbohydrates.

2   Drink liquids between, instead of with, meals.
3   Avoid fatty, fried, or spicy foods, and foods with strong odors.
4   Before going to bed, eat a light snack including both carbohydrates and protein.
5   Before rising, eat a light snack such as soda crackers, dry toasts, or dry cereal.[20]

Constipation is another common complaint in pregnancy, though usually mild. It is caused because hormonal increases in pregnancy decrease peristalsis of the bowel. Again, the client may be advised to follow these suggestions:

1   Increase the fluid intake.
2   Increase the use of natural laxative foods (whole grain, dried fruits).
3   Eat fresh fruits in season.
4   Increase roughage and bulk (raw foods such as lettuce, celery, cabbage).
5   Establish a regular time of day for elimination.[20]

Hemorrhoids, another common complaint, occur because of increased weight and pressure in the abdomen. Previously existing hemorrhoids can be aggravated by this increase in weight and abdominal pressure. Also, constipation will exacerbate the hemorrhoids and cause pain or burning. The nurse should advise her client to do the following:

1   Increase the intake of fluids (up to 14 glasses per day).
2   Chew raw fruits and vegetables thoroughly.[20]

Heartburn or a "full feeling" are also common in pregnancy. The enlargement of the uterus crowds the stomach adjacent to it, and gastric emptying slows down. To help this condition:

1   Reduce the amount of free fat in the diet (fat causes food contents to be retained longer in the stomach).
2   Eat frequent small meals rather than three large meals.
3   Avoid tensions when eating.
4   Drink 3 or 4 ounces of whole milk when the symptom is particularly severe.
5   Avoid preparations containing sodium or sodium bicarbonate.
6   Ask the physician to prescribe antacid preparations.[20]

DIET AND LACTATION

During lactation the mother has special nutritional needs. Her caloric needs increase by 800 to 1000 calories a day, and she should drink at least 1 pint of milk a day. Her calcium and iron requirements are the same as they were when she was pregnant, but she needs more protein (an increase of approximately 65 to 100 grams per day). She also needs to increase her consumption of both A and B vitamin complexes, which are needed for milk production. Obviously, there is an increased need for overall fluid intake, through surprisingly this is often neglected by nursing mothers.[4, 25]

BIBLIOGRAPHY

1   Anderson, L., M. Dibble, H. Mitchell, and H. Rynbergen: *Nutrition in Nursing,* J. B. Lippincott Company, Philadelphia, 1972.

2   Deutsch, Donald M.: *The Family Guide to Better Food and Better Health,* Bantam Books, Inc., New York, 1973.

3   Gutherie, Helen Andrews: *Introductory Nutrition,* The C. V. Mosby Company, St. Louis, 1971.

4*   Williams, Sue Rodwell: *Essentials of Nutrition and Diet Therapy,* The C. V. Mosby Company, St. Louis, 1974.

5*   Mayer, Jean: *A Diet for Living,* David McKay Company, Inc., New York, 1975.

6   Pekkanen, J., and M. Falco: "Sweet and Sour," *Atlantic,* July 1975, pp. 50-53.

7*   *Nutrition Almanac,* Nutrition Search, Inc., McGraw-Hill Book Company, New York, 1975.

8   "Nitrates and Nitrites in Food," *The Medical Letter on Drugs and Therapeutics,* **16**: 75-76, 1974.

9   Magee, P. N.: "Toxicity of Nitrosamines: Their Possible Human Health Hazards," *Food and Cosmetics Toxicology,* **9**: 207-218, 1971.

10   Lijinski, W., et al.: "Carcinogenic Nitrosamines Formed by Drug/Nitrite Interactions," *Nature,* **239**: 165, 1972.

11   Pryde, Lucy T.: *Chemistry of Pesticides, Food and Drugs,* Cummings Publishing Co., Inc., Menlo Park, Calif., 1973.

12   Pyle, James L.: *Chemistry and the Technological Backlash,* Prentice-Hall, Inc., Englewood Cliffs, N.J., 1974.

13   Kermode, G. O.: "Food Additives," *Scientific American,* Mar. 1972, pp. 15-21.

14   Lijinski, W., et al.: "Nitrosation of Tertiary Amines and Some Biologic Implications," *J. Nat. Cancer Inst.,* **439**: 1239-1249, 1972.

15   Shimoda, N.: "Nutrition and Life Style. II. Observations of a Nutritionist in a Free Clinic," *J. Am. Dietetic Assoc.,* **73**: 273-275, 1973.

16   Register, U. D., et al.: "The Vegetarian Diet. Scientific and Practical Considerations," *J. Am. Dietetic Assoc.,* **62**: 253-261, 1973.

17* Lappe, Frances Moore: *Diet for a Small Planet,* rev. ed., Ballantine Books, Inc., New York, 1975.

18* "Vegetarian Diets," *J. Am. Dietetic Assoc.*, **65**: 121-122, 1974.

19   Enstrom, James E.: "Cancer Mortality Among Mormons," *Cancer*, **36** (3): 825-841, 1975.

20* *Nutrition in Pregnancy — Care of the Pregnant Patient*, dev. by The University of Southern California School of Medicine, Raritan, N. J., Omni, Ortho Pharmaceutical Corporation, 1974.

21   Emerson, K., Jr., et al.: "Caloric Cost of Normal Pregnancy," *Obstet. Gynecol.*, **40**: 786-94, 1972.

22   Pitkin, R. M., et al.: "Maternal Nutrition. A Selective Review of Clinical Topics," *Obstet. Gynecol.*, **40**: 773-785, 1972.

23   Wattis, E.: "Eating for Two: The Importance of the Right Type of Food in Pregnancy," *Nursing Times*, **69**: 1248-1249, 1973.

24   Brewer, T. H.: "Human Maternal-Fetal Nutrition," *Obstet. Gynecol.*, **40**: 868-70, 1972.

25   Murry, Ruth, and Judith Zentner: *Nursing Assessment and Health Promotion through the Life Span*, Prentice-Hall, Inc., Englewood Cliffs, N. J., 1975.

26* Church, Charles, and Helen Church: *Food Values of Portions Commonly Used*, J. B. Lippincott Company, Philadelphia, 1975.

27* Crocker, Betty, Pseud.: *Dinner For Two*, Simon and Schuster, New York, 1958.

28* Ewald, Ellen Buchman: *Receipes for a Small Planet*, Ballantine Books, Inc., New York, 1973.

29* Pike, Ruth L., and Myrtle L. Brown: *Nutrition—An Integrated Approach*, 2d ed., John Wiley & Sons, Inc., New York, 1975.

30* White, Philip L., Dean C. Fletcher, and May Ellis: *Nutrients in Processed Foods*, American Medical Association, Publishing Sciences Group, Inc., Acton, Mass., 1975.

*Starred items are of particular interest.

CHAPTER 4

The Sexually Active Young Adult

In no field can the nurse be of more help to her clients than in that of sexuality. In no field should she be more aware of the importance of a completely professional attitude: that is, one which is friendly and encouraging in that she is concerned with the health and well-being of clients, but objective in that it is no business of hers to dictate or pass moral judgment on their life-styles.

In a comparatively short time, there have been in our social view of sexuality so many changes that today the nurse may encounter clients who run the whole gamut of behavior from inhibition to complete permissiveness, who may have little knowledge of facts and much of myths, who are themselves confused and uncertain on a variety of large and small points, and who feel considerable embarrassment in trying to express their difficulties. The primary health care nurse is the ideal person to whom they may turn. She has a background of sound academic preparation. She is at a point of high visibility and availability in the health care delivery system.

Therefore, the first step for the nurse, particularly one in a key setting such as the office of an obstetrician or internist or in an obstetrics and gynecology clinic, is to recognize her professional responsibility and to come to terms with her own attitudes and feelings. In this way she can become comfortable and can make her

51

clients comfortable as they discuss sexuality together. A second step is for the nurse to become very knowledgeable in the area of normal human sexual behavior. A review of current research findings is an appropriate way to begin.

MALE AND FEMALE: SIMILARITIES AND DIFFERENCES

Beginning with the Kinsey Report, there has been considerable research on the sexual behavior of the American adult. The data reveal some conflicting information about the similarities and differences between men and women. Aside from their obvious anatomical differences, other characteristics have been studied, such as response to explicit sexual stimuli, age at which peak of sexual activity is reached, and inclination towards variety in sex.

There has been a great deal of speculation and joking about the periodicity of a woman's emotions and sexual drive as related to her menstrual cycle. The frequency of sexual activity for women tends to vary except for a reported depression during the luteal phase of the cycle.[1] Some researchers conclude that progesterone is responsible and that its presence during natural cycles affects the male so that he does not desire coitus as frequently during the luteal phase. They postulate that the influence on the male may operate via a *pheromone*, a distinctive odor, as is the case with other male mammals.[2]

Other researchers maintain that the effect of hormonal fluctuations on female sexual behavior is highly idiosyncratic, with environmental, cultural, and cognitive variables being much more potent.[3,4] White women reach their peak of sexual responsiveness and activity in their late thirties and early forties.[5] Freed from the possibility of pregnancy by the arrival of menopause or by sterilization, they either remain at a plateau or may report an increase in interest and frequency of sexual experience.[5,6] White men, on the other hand, reach their sexual peak before the age of 20 and experience a gradual decline in their interest and activity as they become more absorbed in work, business, or professional activities.[5] Marked incongruity in the sexual cycles of two partners will potentially be a source of conflict unless ways are found to meet the needs of both without exploiting one or the other. We will consider this issue further when we look at the sexual ramifications of pregnancy.

The Kinsey data suggest that men are sexually aroused by pictures of nude women, sex jokes, erotic stories, and music that has erotic overtones, while women are more likely to respond to love stories, poetry, and romantic scenes in movies. Subsequent research, however, has shown that adults of both sexes in their twenties exhibit similar patterns and intensity of reactions to explicit sexual stimuli, such as erotic stories and pictures of nudes.[7]

SEXUAL BEHAVIOR

According to Schmidt, today's young adults have a traditional view of sexuality—that is, women behave sexually as if they had less sexual drive than men; show fewer signs of frustration when they abstain sexually; behave as though they should show less sexual initiative than their male partner, or at least not more than he; and behave as if their sexuality is more dependent on love, personal relations, and fidelity than is men's.[8] However, during the last 10 to 15 years, there has been a convergent trend resulting in a steady decline of these sex differences. An overwhelming majority of young men and women now have permissive and egalitarian sex standards.[9-11] A pattern of "coitus with commitment" for males as well as females is beginning to emerge,[12] and the formality of an engagement does not seem to be an important condition.[13] The incidence of premarital necking and petting and of premarital coitus is equally high for men and women.

Sexual intercouse is perceived by many of both sexes in America today as having value not only for its procreative possibilities but for other reasons as well: it meets the needs for body contact and for physical expression of the sex drive; it is used to express trust, love, and affection; and it reaffirms an integral part of an individual's self concept. Premarital sex means less use by the woman of her body as bait in the matrimonial trap and should be good preparation for better marriage, if and when it occurs. Women are as ready as men to experiment with more than one partner. Unmarried men and women are demonstrating an increased capacity to enter into coital relations without feelings of guilt and/or remorse. Differences regarding the incidence of masturbation have decreased considerably, although men still demonstrate a higher incidence than women.[14-17]

However, although we are supposedly living in an era of sexual enlightenment and increasing sexual freedom, in some key matters young adults are still asserting traditional values. They continue to judge the appropriateness of relationships in terms of the social categories of the partners, such as gender (i.e., homosexual versus heterosexual lovers), age, class, and race. They are concerned with the social relationship between the partners; namely, are they single, married to each other, or married to someone else? The number of sex partners at a given time is also of concern. But probably the most important single element in the formation of an opinion is the consequence of the behavior; sexual intercourse which transmits venereal disease or causes an unwanted pregnancy is generally unacceptable.

CONTRACEPTION

Many would agree that the person who is old enough to be sexually active is old enough to take responsibility for conception control. Information about the nature, efficacy, side effects, and contraindications of contraceptive devices available are well described elsewhere. Some comments on the effects of the various methods on sex relations is in order.

Rhythm Since the rhythm method is an integral part of the life-style of some couples, it may not have an appreciable effect on their sex relations. However, for some, the rhythm method hampers spontaneity. Most couples find it difficult to refrain from sexual relations for the length of time needed to be safe.

Condom If the couple is comfortable enough with each other to make the putting on of the condom a part of their sex play, it should have no effect. Some men say that wearing a condom interferes with full sexual pleasure, but some women say that this position is a "cop-out" for accepting shared responsibility for conception control.

Contraceptive Foam Some people resist using a contraceptive before each new sex act. Otherwise, foam does not interfere with either partner's pleasure.

Diaphragm If it is properly fitted and inserted, neither partner generally feels the diaphragm during intercourse. Some women, especially those who have trouble comfortably touching their genitalia, do not like to insert and remove it, so it may affect their attitude towards the sex act. Some women are able to enjoy intercourse during menstruation because they use the diaphragm to temporarily dam the menstrual flow.

Intrauterine Device When properly inserted, it is felt by neither partner. It may increase enjoyment indirectly because it relieves anxiety over possible pregnancy.

Oral Contraceptive Since anxiety over possible pregnancy is reduced, there is probably an indirect effect on pleasure experienced during the sex act. Some research currently appearing in the literature indicates that loss of libido may be a side effect for some women on oral contraceptives.[18] Masters and Johnson report a few cases of sexual dysfunction attributable to women taking "the pill." Usually, the women had been using oral contraceptives for 18 months to 3 years and the dysfunction was reversible simply by taking them off the pill.[19] Grant and Mears[20] found that women taking highly progestogenic contraceptive pills were far more apt to complain of loss of libido than those taking highly estrogenic preparations. Other research has found this difference to be insignificant.[21]

PERSONAL HYGIENE

Young adults should maintain good genital health in the same way as they maintain good dental health—with regular cleaning and periodic checkups. The genitalia, like the mouth, have certain qualities which make them at once vulnerable and yet strangely resistant to disease organisms. A number of simple precautions can be taken by the adult to maintain good personal hygiene and discourage an environment conducive to growing pathogens. Nurses should be prepared to offer this information without being asked.

Men should be advised to use a pure soap like Ivory for washing the genitalia, since regular, frequent use of deodorant or antibacterial soaps can remove natural oils and cause dry skin. They should pay special attention to crevices, and if uncircumcised, to the area under the foreskin.

Women should use plain warm water to remove all excess vaginal secretions. Their sweetish odor changes as the secretions move to the outside and are exposed to the air, but strong odors are probably due to an infection, which will need treatment. Deodorant soaps and antibacterial detergents remove natural oils and bacteria that are necessary for keeping the vagina and outer genitalia healthy. Use of a pure soap on the pubic hair and outer lips is recommended. Some women prefer to keep their pubic hair clipped short to cut down on odors from dried urine. Other women find that wearing cotton underpants or synthetic underpants with a cotton crotch decreases feelings of moistness and discomfort, since cotton "breathes" better than the synthetics and allows for absorption and evaporation due to some amount of airflow. Bubble bath products may be very irritating to the genitalia. A douche each month after the menstrual period to remove old cells is probably not harmful, but frequent douching upsets the natural balance of the vaginal flora, predisposing the woman to infection. Disinfectant douches and feminine hygiene sprays may contain ingredients irritating to the sensitive skin of vagina and labia. They are expensive and unnecessary. Women who insist on douching should avoid the bulb-squeeze syringe and other pressure devices for forcing fluids into the vagina (or inadvertently into the abdomen). A generally safe solution to use is 4 tablespoons of white distilled vinegar in 2 quarts of water.

Both men and women, whenever possible, should wash the anal area after a bowel movement instead of merely wiping with toilet paper. Women should wipe from front to back so as not to carry any bacteria from the anus to the openings of the vagina or urethra.

PREMARITAL PHYSICAL EXAM

VIGNETTE
Eva is early for her premarital physical exam. She asks the office nurse if they might talk privately for a few minutes. In the conversation that ensues, she confesses to some feelings of rejection by her fiance since, immediately following intercourse, he goes to the bathroom to wash his genitalia. She asks if there is anything abnormal about his behavior.

Regardless of the wealth of material that has recently been published and the frequency of open discussion of sexuality on radio and television, the issue of normalcy continues to trouble many young adults. One cannot conclude that individuals will freely discuss their sexual behavior with others in an attempt to validate the normalcy of certain aspects of it. On the contrary, the more uncertain an individual is about a behavior, the less likely he is to bring it out in the open.

One working definition of normal has been proposed by Chez: "Whatever is pleasurable and gratifying for both participants is normal for that couple as long as there is communication and mutual participation without coercion."[22] If people are comfortable with this definition, it allows much more leeway in their behavior than if they cling to a definition having its roots in religious or common law or personal preference. It is wise to remember that there remain a few individuals who define their own behavior as normal and anything different as abnormal or deviant.

The issue of her fiance's hygiene seems an insignificant matter, but it has troubled Eva for months. She perceived it as indication that she was somehow unclean, or that her vaginal secretions were repulsive. The nurse encouraged Eva to share her feelings with her fiance and to explore with him the meaning of his behavior. The nurse further emphasized the importance of establishing a habit of honest, open communication about their sexual experience as a strong foundation for their marriage. The sexual part of a committed relationship is particularly vulnerable to invasion by false assumptions and hurt or angry feelings. One of the most important preventive nursing measures is to stress the need for honest exchange of feelings, and the need for checking out with the partner how things are going with him.

Although nurses in the past have been socialized to refrain from any exchange of personal information with a patient, in this instance it would probably be therapeutic. For example the nurse might tell her client that her own husband customarily goes into the kitchen and fixes himself a snack after intercourse. The nurse's role modeling as she recounts this part of her sexual pattern will demonstrate to Eva that a sense of humor can put things into perspective and reduce some of her anxiety. While it may be true that Eva could get this kind of advice and support from a friend, the primary health care nurse must accept sexual counseling of this nature as a part of her professional responsibility.

The occasion of the premarital exam is an excellent opportunity to set the climate for a discussion of sexual concerns, either then or at some later time. Research has shown that young people overwhelmingly express a desire for the physician to offer contraceptive and sexual counseling during the premarital exam. A typical comment was

> I want the physician to tell me specifically about sexual adjustment. I might be too embarrassed to ask if he does not volunteer such information. I want him not just to say that sex is normal and good. I want to know about frequency, differences in desire between males and females, about orgasm, about potency, and impotency, and about how to make sexual life good for both of us.[23]

There is no reason why nurses could not provide some of this health education. In reality, many are probably better prepared than the physician for the responsibility of transmitting both accurate information and healthy attitudes. Of the respondents in the above research, a large majority preferred conjoint exams and a discussion of the results of the physical exam and counseling about sexual adjustment and contraceptive techniques with both partners.

Anticipatory guidance can also be offered to the young adult woman who is more or less sexually inexperienced. Catapulted into an extended sexual exposure, she runs a high risk of developing "honeymoonitis," a condition in which prolonged friction of the genitals may traumatize the urinary meatus, which then becomes contaminated with normal vaginal bacteria, resulting in cystitis. The condition responds easily to drug therapy, although the woman may feel chagrined at seeking treatment unless she understands that it is an autoinfection, and not a disease brought to her by her new husband.

Nurses should be aware of what is published in lay magazines about sexual behavior. Readers may be left with the impression that there is no room for individual variation. For example, a young man may mistakenly label himself "over the hill" because he is 30. The adult who has been led by what he hears and reads to believe that his sexual performance should match some national norm is either setting himself up for failure or may feel that he is leading an unimaginative, unexciting sexual existence. Nurses have the responsibility to provide patients with access to correct information and to help them feel comfortable with a pattern of sexual activity uniquely suited to the needs and desires of both partners in the relationship.

THE SEX HISTORY

One of the vehicles for providing sexual counseling is the sex history. There is some difference of opinion as to whether or not it is either necessary or appropriate to take a complete sexual history on the occasion of the premarital exam. It is, however, a highly appropriate time to obtain the baseline sexual data at this milestone of a couple's life. If the couple has been sexually active for considerable time, some of the data may already be known to the health care team. Though it is sometimes assumed that the sexually experienced individual does not need basic sex education, this assumption is not safe. The routine inclusion of questions about sexual knowledge and experience can defuse some of the issues which commonly generate anxiety in clients. Taking a sexual history provides an opportunity to give the client information and reassurance as well as to identify gaps and errors in his knowledge. From the baseline data, a management plan can be formulated, implemented, and evaluated. If the issues which surface are beyond the scope of competence of the nurse, the client can immediately be referred to the appropriate professional or agency without having to wait until the problem is of such magnitude that it has devastated the lives of the couple involved.

Several rules of thumb will help the interviewer reduce the client's inevitable anxiety.

1   Provide privacy for the interview and insure confidentiality of information.
2   Ask the client how he or she acquired sexual information before you ask about the experience.
3   Use common rather than technical language—the client will feel more comfortable responding in terms he or she knows or uses.
4   Progress from topics easy to discuss to those more difficult.

5 Let the client resolve this own moral questions and define what is normal for himself.

6 During the interview, precede questions with informational statements about the generality of the experience; it will help to reduce the client's shame, anxiety, and evasiveness.

The content of the sex history should include details of early sexual training and experience, family attitudes towards sex, amount of demonstrativeness in the home, personal attitudes toward sex, the significance of sex within past and current relationships, sexual preferences, and any sex-related traumas.

Because of the acutely sensitive nature of the information, only minimal writing should be done during the interview. The client's anxiety will escalate if she or he is distracted by the nurse's strict adherence to a printed form or copious note taking. It is rarely essential that all available information be recorded after only one interview, and areas that are unclear or overlooked can be picked up on subsequent visits. In fact, it is often a comfortable entree to resume discussion of a sensitive area with a point of clarification from a previous interview. (See sexual history tool, Chapter 16.)

SEXUALITY AND CHILDBEARING

Since women are endowed biologically with the capacity to bear children, we shall assume that pregnancy in and of itself does not constitute a significant departure from a state of general good health unless there are medical complications for either the mother or the fetus. Pregnancy, then, is a variation in a state of health to which almost all women are at risk, especially during early adulthood when statistically they are most likely to be sexually active. Consequently, it merits attention here for its impact on the sexual life of the woman and her mate.

It is safe to assume that most pregnant women want information concerning the physiological and emotional aspects of sexual activity during pregnancy. Many inhibitions surround most clients' disclosures of experiences and feelings in this area, so it is wise for the nurse to be well informed about normal variation in sexuality at different points during pregnancy. The normative data described below can supply a sound basis of fact for nurses counseling pregnant couples.

Much is known about endocrine changes associated with both the normal menstrual cycle and the experience of pregnancy. Researchers have demonstrated interest in the possible interrelationship of hormonal levels and the woman's sex drive. Some knowledge and considerable speculation has been generated by the studies reported. Since direct observation of sexual behavior by the investigator is generally impossible, subjects are asked to report feelings and experiences either by completing a questionnaire or by being interviewed. There is always the possibility of incomplete or inaccurate recall, especially if the behavior in question occurred several months before.

A study on a number of human cultures, conducted by Ford and Beach,[24] reports considerable prohibition of female sexual activity during pregnancy. Of sixty societies reported, twenty-one, or about 30 percent, prohibit sex relations from the second months of pregnancy and 50 percent from the sixth month on. Of the twenty-one, nineteen recognize other legitimate sexual outlets for the husband. The authors note that the taboo is usually explained as an attempt to prevent fetal injury.

One of the best known studies of sex during pregnancy has been done by Masters and Johnson.[25] In their research laboratory, they observed and measured the sexual function of six pregnant women ranging in age from 21 to 36. In general, the women's sexual responses were physiologically the same as those of nonpregnant women, with the exception of some increased breast tenderness, a heightened arousal during the second trimester, and a slightly longer resolution phase following orgasm. Regular verbal reports from another group of 101 women as their pregnancies progressed revealed the following general pattern: the same degree of sexual desire and functioning in the first trimester as before pregnancy, an increase in the second, and a decrease in the third. The researchers suggest that third trimester results may have been due to the fact that about 47 percent of the women had been warned by their doctor to avoid intercourse for at least part of the time. They further report a range of delay of return to sexual desire after childbirth from 2 to 3 weeks to over 3 months. The twenty-four mothers in their study who were breastfeeding indicated a prompter return of sexuality and a return to higher levels of functioning than the others. Sexual arousal was the occasion of "deep guilt feelings" in twelve of these mothers.

In opposition to the Masters and Johnson findings, Solberg, Butler, and Wagner[26] report a linear decrease in sexual activity, interest, and noncoital *pregnant* behavior in American women. In their study, coital frequency at all stages of pregnancy was independent of race, religious preference, male or female level of education, negative feelings about being pregnant, and whether or not the pregnancy was planned. Of the 260 women interviewed, only 5 (2 percent) received recommendations from their physicians or other paramedical personnel concerning sexual activities that might be substituted for coitus during pregnancy. Ten percent received recommendations about positions that might be more comfortable, with side-by-side or rear entry being most common. Twenty-nine percent received instructions recommending coital abstention, but only 8 percent claimed to have directly changed their behavior as a result of physician's instructions. Women who experienced a negative change in degree or intensity of their sexual experience during pregnancy reported physical discomfort, fear of injury to the baby, awkwardness having coitus, and perceived loss of attractiveness as additional reasons in their own minds for the change. The reported general decrease in noncoital behavior such as masturbation, hand-stimulation by the partner, and mutual oral-genital stimulation suggests that, in addition to attitudes and comfort with sexuality, a biological factor may be involved in the declining frequency. It is important to remember that there was considerable individual variation reported by the women in the study related to their interest and activity in both coital and noncoital behavior. Nurses interested in delivering individually determined client care must bear in mind the unique and highly individualistic nature of sexual feelings.

Falicov[27] gathered data which indicated that on the whole, subjects had positive attitudes toward sexual intercourse during the pregnancy and valued sexual expression as a form of marital communication, yet they all experienced a general decrease in sexual involvement. Like the Masters and Johnson data, there was some increase in coital frequency and satisfaction during the second trimester, but it continued to be below prepregnancy levels.

In the Kenny[28] studies, almost half of all the subjects reported a resumption of sexual interest earlier than 4 weeks after delivery, a phenomenon which corroborates Masters and Johnson's findings that there was a prompter return of sexual desire and a return to higher levels of sexual functioning among breastfeeding women than among nonbreastfeeders. Kenny points out, however, that his sample is unusual in that breastfeeding mothers are still in a minority and tend to cluster in certain social classes in our society.

Controversy continues over whether or not sexual activity during late pregnancy and premature birth are correlated. Javert[29] contended that frequent or multiple orgasm early in pregnancy might precipitate an abortion, whereas Pugh and Fernandez[30] found no relation between the two variables. Goodlin estimated a 15 percent prematurity risk factor for women continuing to be orgasmic after 32 weeks.[31] However, in the Solberg study[26] the prematurity rate of women who had orgasm after the seventh month was less than 6 percent and not significantly different from the rest of his sample.

In addition to birth weight and gestational age at delivery, APGAR scores at 1 minute were also independent of either frequency of coitus or rate of orgasm during the last trimester of pregnancy.

Lack of knowledge about normal sexual changes during pregnancy and postpartum causes women considerable anxiety about the normalcy of their reactions. The nurse must be ready to volunteer information and encourage communication on the topic. This is particularly reassuring during the early months of pregnancy, when few women are likely to anticipate a diminution of sexual drive.

Clients who are concerned about some aspect of their sexuality yet reluctant to bring it up for discussion, may send out very subtle signals to the nurse in the hope that he or she will pick up and decode their message. The nurse may perceive an attitude of "holding back" in a client and may ask, "Is there anything else you would like to discuss?" Nonverbal behavior—posture, tone of voice, a gesture—can also give the nurse a clue to unfinished business. The client may invite the nurse into further conversation with seemingly unrelated comments such as "I hope there's no such thing as a 12-month baby" or "I feel like a nun!" The nurse must ascertain what the client is really trying to communicate and not simply brush her off with a good-natured laugh and a "There, there. You'll feel different when it's all over" attitude.

Because fear of harming the fetus seems to be an almost universal phenomenon, the nurse or the physician should be prepared to explain what is currently known about the precise mechanism whereby the fetus can be affected, either directly by the various positions assumed during sexual intercourse or indirectly by transmission of diseases or premature rupture of membranes. For couples who seem to have difficulty imagining unfamiliar positions, simple sketches are helpful to show how legs and bodies can be arranged. Some couples may equate rear entry with bestiality or sodomy and require extra teaching and reassurance (or permission) that this position is an appropriate alternative to male or female superior.

As well as information about positions, alternative expressions of sexuality and their meaning to each partner need to be explored.

VIGNETTE

Carol is 8 months pregnant with her first child. Although active and healthy, she is beginning to feel awkward and clumsy, and experiences some shortness of breath in certain sitting and lying positions. She is aware that her sex drive is reduced from her prepregnant state. On the one hand, she is secretly grateful that her husband, Nick, places few demands on her; but on the other hand, she feels a responsibility to help him gain release for his sexual tension. After several weeks of his not approaching her, Carol initiates fellatio, oral-genital sex, a practice which Nick craves but she does not enjoy.

On her next visit to the obstetrician, Carol confides to the office nurse that having never experienced it before, she is repulsed by the taste, odor, and feel of the semen. She asks the nurse about ways to help her better participate in this type of sexual expression.

Since Carol obviously wants to try to give pleasure to her mate, some very practical hints are in order. Since absolute cleanliness of the genitalia will eliminate stale body and urine odors, she can encourage Nick to shower immediately before sexual activity or incorporate a warm soapy facecloth and towel into her own sex play. Another alternative would be for them to shower together, using that opportunity to engage in touching and caressing. Assuming the superior position will allow Carol to control the thrusting so that she does not gag. She should be encouraged to be honest with Nick about her feelings and enlist his support for a gradual progression from mere fondling of his penis to ejaculation, or consider fellatio and masturbation together as a possible alternative. Knowledge of some basic facts about the composition, harmlessness, and sterility of normal ejaculate might help her in overcoming her repulsion.

Considering that prolonged prohibition of intercourse may lead to feelings of estrangement between the partners, the nurse should provide anticipatory guidance to couples who ask about safe limits. Sexual intercourse should stop if it causes vaginal or abdominal pain or in the presence of any type of uterine bleeding (indicating possible abortion in the first trimester or placenta previa in the third trimester). All genital sex play should stop once the membranes have ruptured, to prevent the possibility of infection. When sexual intercourse is prohibited by the physician because of the possibility of inducing abortion, the woman should also refrain from masturbation to the point of orgasm, since uterine contractions occur in each case.

Following delivery, sexual intercouse may be safely resumed when bleeding has ceased and there is relatively no perineal discomfort. Anxiety about this resumption may be related to fear of soreness caused by the episiotomy, physical discomfort because of engorged breasts, or changes perceived in the woman's sexual organs—vaginal muscles may seem either tighter making intercourse painful, or stretched, a condition women fear may detract from the male's sexual enjoyment. On the other hand, because of the greater vasocongestion in the postpartum pelvis, women may experience greater orgasmic capacity than before the pregnancy.

Breastfeeding mothers should be further advised that the hypothalmic portion of the brain does not discriminate between sources of breast stimulation. The same nerve pathways carry the impulse, regardless of whether it results from an infant sucking or a mate kissing the nipples. During periods of sexual arousal, therefore, it is common for the breasts to leak. Couples who are not prepared for this experience may be shocked, annoyed, or amused, depending on their state of mind. Mothers who experience sexual arousal when their infants nurse may feel less guilty if they understand it to be a physiological response over which they have no control. They will do best if they can relax and enjoy the good feelings.

SEXUALITY AND CHILDREARING

The nurse in the pediatrician's office may also find herself in a position to counsel the young adult in the area of sexuality, as evidenced in the following vignette.

VIGNETTE

Alan and Betty are a young couple with a preschool son. Alan's job requires him to leave the house at 5 A.M. each morning; Betty's job begins later in the morning and she frequently doesn't arrive home until 5:30 or 6:00 P.M. Consequently their sleep patterns are different and their sex life has become routinized to mainly weekend episodes. One afternoon, in an effort to introduce some variety, they escape to their bedroom while their preschooler is involved watching "Sesame Street." Sex play is short, and during intercourse Betty is tense and watchful, expecting the child to burst in at any moment. He does precisely that. Curious, but not unnerved by the sight of his parents in their missionary position, he seems satisfied by Alan's explanation that "Daddy is just hugging Mommy" and is distracted by an invitation to join them—on top of, rather than under the sheets—for a tickling session. After a few minutes, he returns to his program and Alan thrusts on to ejaculation. Betty is inorgasmic, and for days after the incident she struggles with some feelings of guilt regarding its possible effect on her son.

A few weeks later, during a routine visit to the pediatrician, Betty hesitantly asks the nurse about the effect on children of observing their parents engaging in sexual intercourse.

The alert primary health care nurse will support Betty and Alan in their efforts to continue to work at and enrich their own sexual relationship. The nurse can also point out that children learn what they experience far better than what they are told. The day-to-day role modeling of affectionate parents constitutes a most significant part of the children's sex education. Children can learn that parents need "private" time—whether it be to read, meditate, make love, or whatever. They will understand this better if parents afford them the same privilege. Each family can work out its own signals for identifying a member's need to be alone. When children are old enough to read, it might be a "Do Not Disturb" sign on the door. Until then, Alan and Betty might well consider buying a lock for their bedroom. If that is not an acceptable possibility, the nurse might suggest that they barricade the door temporarily with a piece of furniture like a dresser or heavy chair.

Betty is probably having guilt feelings about leaving her preschooler unsupervised while she and Alan have intercourse. It is true that Betty will not relax and enjoy the experience with her husband if she is worried about her son. On the other hand, concern about children is a handy excuse for avoiding intercourse. The nurse can help her realistically think through ways to safeguard the child's environment or pre-plan her sexual encounters so that they may occur at a time when he is either asleep or under someone else's supervision. The nurse may have to help Betty to deal with the myth that spontaneous sex is superior. The spur-of-the-moment stop at the local hamburger stand for supper and the carefully prepared gourmet dinner are both forms of eating; each is highly appropriate and extremely pleasurable in its own way, depending on the circumstances of the moment and the preferences of the people involved. It is important that Betty and Alan be as ingenious as possible at maintaining their sexual relationship, since it adds zest to their present living and is an excellent safeguard against loss of interest and declining satisfaction as the years progress. Perhaps the most helpful thing the nurse can do is give Betty permission to engage in behaviors designed to enrich her sexual life and thereby her marriage.

ALTERNATE LIFE-STYLES

The simple fact of choosing an alternate life-style does not constitute a problem about which nursing needs to concern itself. However, the implications of that choice may include situations in the sexual experience of the individual which lend themselves to some anticipatory guidance from the nurse. Sexually transmitted disease is a health hazard to which all sexually active people are vulnerable. And dealing with a health care delivery system which is basically heterosexual becomes a major issue for the person who has a homosexual preference.

Involvement in premarital or extramarital sexual relationships, especially if multiple partners are involved, includes the possibility of exposure to sexually transmitted diseases. Much has been written about the etiology and treatment of both gonorrhea and syphilis, but the reality of the present is that the less-known diseases such as herpes simplex type II and venereal warts are becoming increasingly common and are every bit as troublesome.

In 1975, the New York Alliance for the Eradication of Venereal Diseases, Inc., published a pamphlet containing some helpful suggestions for preventing sexually transmitted disease.[32] They recommend that immediately after intercourse, the male should soap his genitals, working some of the suds into the urinary meatus. He should rinse, repeat the procedure and then urinate (which may sting). Extended exposure or delay before washing diminishes effectiveness of this preventive measure. If lubricants are used during sexual intercourse, they should be water-soluble rather than oil-base preparations so that they will wash away and not leave a film to trap pathogens. The condom is a highly effective method of prevention, tracing its origin to the sixteenth century. Condoms are made of latex or especially processed animal membrane and are available dry or prelubricated. They should be placed over the erect penis before contact or penetration, leaving a small pouch at the tip to collect the semen, and should be removed before the penis becomes flaccid again. The male should grasp the open end of the condom to minimize the possibility of it slipping off during withdrawal of the penis from the vagina.

Probably because of the nature of the female anatomy, there is very little in the literature about specific preventive measures for the female. At a recent convention in Chicago, the American Medical Association's House of Delegates endorsed as preventative measures against gonorrhea "abstinence" for the single person and "fidelity and continence" for married couples. Neither of these options may seem reasonable for some women. Urinating after having intercourse and thorough regular cleansing of the genitalia are sound general preventive measures, but the sad reality is that most women with VD don't know it until it is diagnosed. The nurse should advise the heterosexually active women to buy her own supply of condoms and insist that her sexual partner wear one. Obviously the reporting, tracing, and treatment of contacts is another critical preventive health measure.

If we can agree that all consenting adults have a right to their own sexual orientation and preferences, how can the nurse convey a respectful attitude to clients whose life-style is not that of the majority? Questions can be phrased to inquire about "sexual partners," not a girlfriend or a boyfriend. Clients should be routinely offered diagnostic tests involving mouth, throat, and anus rather than having to request them. It should not be assumed that all women automatically need conception information, since it presupposes that they have a heterosexual relationship. Neither should the nurse imply that there is something irresponsible about denying the need for contraceptive information. If the couple is lesbian, they simply aren't at risk for an unwanted pregnancy. The nurse should never assume that the homosexual client is a misguided heterosexual or that he regrets his sexual preference. Couples or women who have made an informed choice not to have children also have the right to be taken seriously. A disbelieving nurse will simply alienate them or drive them to another health care facility. Similarly, monogamy is not for every person. Some perfectly normal young adults choose to remain single, experiment with group marriage, or live with a lover. They have a right to their choice.

Clients need assurance that their health record will be kept confidential because they may fear that information will be used against them, e.g., regarding employment or promotion opportunities. Above all, the nurse must realize that when false assumptions about sexual behavior are made, the door to open communication often slams shut. The nurse should strive to use neutral terms when discussing human sexuality with a patient, to give choices, and to leave those choices open. The empathic nurse has the potential to act as a catalyst to allow the client to express himself more fully as a sexual person and to be treated in a respectful, nonjudgmental way.

This chapter has reviewed what is currently known about sexual differences between men and women, normative changes which have occurred over the past 10 to 15 years, and sexual behavior in the young adult. Childbearing and child rearing are examined because they are major stressors on the sexual health of young married adults and they are developmental tasks most commonly found in, but not limited to, this age group. Considerable focus seems to have been placed on alternate life-styles. It would be irresponsible to leave the reader with the impression that these life-styles are found only in young adults. They have been considered here for reasons of convenience only. The reader should assume that health issues associated with alternative life-styles are common across the life cycle with minor variations related to age.

BIBLIOGRAPHY
1   Udry, J. Richard, and Naomi M. Morris: "Distribution of Coitus in the Menstrual Cycle," *Nature*, **220** (5167): 593-596, 1968.

2   Udry, J. Richard, Naomi M. Morris, and Lynn Waller: "Effects of Contraceptive Pills on Sexual Activity in the Luteal Phase of the Human Menstrual Cycle," *Arch. Sexual Behavior*, 2 (3): 205-214, 1973.

3   Griffith, Mac, and C. Eugene Walker: "Menstrual Cycle Phases and Personality Variables as Related to Response to Erotic Stimuli," *Arch. Sexual Behavior*, 4 (6): 599-603, 1975.

4   Spitz, Cathy J., Alice R. Gold, and David B. Adams: "Cognitive and Hormonal Factors Affecting Coital Frequency," *Arch. of Sexual Behavior*, 4 (3): 249-263, 1975.

5   Kaplan, H. S.: *The New Sex Therapy*. Brunner/Mazel, Inc., New York, 1974.

6   Brecher, Ruth, and Edward Brecher: *An Analysis of Human Sexual Response*, pp. 88—96, Signet Books, New American Library, Inc., New York, 1966.

7   Schmidt, Gunter: "Male-Female Differences in Sexual Arousal and Behavior During and After Exposure to Sexually Explicit Stimuli," *Arch. Sexual Behavior*, 4 (4): 353-365, 1975.

8   Schmidt, Gunter, and Volkmar Sigusch: "Changes in Sexual Behavior Among Young Males and Females Between 1960-1970," *Arch. Sexual Behavior*, 2 (1): 27-45, 1972.

9   Smigel, E. O., and R. Seiden: "The Decline and Fall of the Double Standard," *Ann. Am. Acad. Political Social Sci.*, 376: 6-17, 1968.

10 Bell, R. R.: *Premarital Sex in a Changing Society*, Prentice-Hall, Inc., Englewood Cliffs, N.J. 1966.

11 Reiss, I. L.: "The Sexual Renaissance in America: a Summary and Analysis," *J. Social Issues*, 22: 123-137, 1966.

12 Lewis, Robert A., and Wesley R. Burr: "Premarital Coitus and Commitment Among College Students," *Arch. Sexual Behavior*, 4 (1): 73-79, 1975.

13 Bell, R. R., and J. B. Chaskes: "Premarital Sexual Experience Among Coeds, 1958-1968," *J. Marriage Family*, 32: 81-84, 1970.

14 Pope, H., and D. D. Knudsen: "Premarital Sexual Norms, the Family, and Social Change," *J. Marriage Family*, 27: 314-323, 1965.

15 Christensen, H. T., and C. F. Gregg: "Changing Sex Norms in America and Scandinavia," *J. Marriage Family*, 32: 616-627, 1970.

16 Kaats, G. R., and K. E. Davis: "The Dynamics of Sexual Behavior of College Students," *J. Marriage Family*, 32: 390-399, 1970.

17 Hunt, Morton: *Sexual Behavior in the 1970's*, Playboy Press, Chicago, 1974.

18 Herzberg, Brenda N., Katharine C. Draper, Anthony L. Johnson, and Gillian C. Nicol: "Oral Contraceptives, Depression, and Libido," *Brit. Med. J.*, 3: 495-500, 1971.

19 Masters, William: "Human Sexuality," Lecture delivered at workshop at Oasis Midwest Center for Human Potential, Chicago, May 19, 1974.

20 Grant, Ellen, and Eleanor Mears: "Mental Effects of Oral Contraceptives," *Lancet*, II: 945-946, 1967.

21 Udry, J. Richard, and Naomi M. Morris: "Effect of Contraceptive Pills on the Distribution of Sexual Activity in the Menstrual Cycle," *Nature*, 227 (5257): 502-503, 1970.

22   Chez, R. A.: "The Female Patient's Sexual History," in C. W. Wahl (ed.), *Sexual Problems: Diagnosis and Treatment in Medical Practice*, The Free Press, New York, 1967.

23   Nash, Ethel M., and Lois M. Louden: "The Premarital Medical Examination and the Carolina Population Center: What Patients Desire," *J. Am. Med. Assoc.* **210** (13): 2365-2369, 1969.

24   Ford, O. S., and F. A. Beach: *Patterns of Sexual Behavior*, Perennial Library, Harper & Row, Publishers, Incorporated, New York, 1951.

25   Masters, William, and Virginia Johnson: *Human Sexual Response*, pp. 141-168, Little, Brown and Company, Boston, 1966.

26   Solberg, Don A., Julius Butler, and Nathaniel N. Wagner: "Sexual Behavior in Pregnancy," *N. Engl. J. Med.*, **288** (21): 1098-1103, 1973.

27   Falicov, Celia J.: "Sexual Adjustment During First Pregnancy and Post Partum," *Am. J. Obstet. Gynecol.*, **117** (7): 991-1000, 1973.

28   Kenny, James A.: "Sexuality of Pregnant and Breastfeeding Women," *Arch. Sexual Behavior*, **3**: 215-229, 1973.

29   Javert, C. T.: *Spontaneous and Habitual Abortion*, McGraw-Hill Book Company, New York, 1957.

30   Pugh, W. E., and F. L. Fernandez: "Coitus in Late Pregnancy: a Follow-up Study of the Effects of Coitus on Late Pregnancy, Delivery and the Puerperium," *Obstet. Gynecol.*, **2**: 636-642, 1953.

31   Goodlin, R. C., D. W. F. Keller, and M. Raffin: "Orgasm During Late Pregnancy: Possible Deleterior Effects," *Obstet. Gynecol.*, **38**: 916-920, 1971.

32   "Venereal Disease Prevention for Everyone," New York Alliance for the Eradication of Venereal Disease, Inc., New York, 1975.

33*   Boston Women's Health Book, Collective: *Our Bodies, Ourselves*, Simon and Schuster, New York, 1976.

34*   Butler, Julius C., and Nathaniel N. Wagner: "Sexuality During Pregnancy and Post-Partum," in *Human Sexuality: A Health Practitioner's Text*, pp. 133-144, The Williams & Wilkins Company, Baltimore, 1975.

35*   Cherniak, Donna, and Allan Feingold: *VD Handbook*, Montreal Health Press, Inc., Montreal, 1972.

36   *Catalog of Sexual Consciousness:* Saul Braun (ed.), Grove Press, Inc., New York, 1975.

37*   Dodson, Betty: *Liberating Masturbation: a Meditation on Self Love*, Bodysex Designs, New York, 1974.

38*   Green, Richard: "Taking a Sex History," in *Human Sexuality: A Health Practitioner's Text*, p. 9-19, The Williams & Wilkins Company, Baltimore, 1975.

39*   Secondi, John J.: *For People Who Make Love: a Guide to Sexual Health*, Bantam Books, Inc., New York, 1974.

40*   Woods, Nancy Fugate: *Human Sexuality in Health and Illness*, pp. 59-75, The C. V. Mosby Company, St. Louis, 1975.

*Starred items are of particular interest.

CHAPTER 5

Environmental Health

The environment surrounds us today with hidden dangers our ancestors never knew. We grow up with strontium 90 in our bones, dichlorodiphenyltrichloroethane (DDT) in our fat, and asbestos in our lungs.[1] We are confronted with vast amounts of conflicting information about these dangers, and it is difficult to know what to believe — particularly for the nurse, who has the responsibility of providing anticipatory guidance. Isolated bits of information, such as the statement that one chemical has been proven carcinogenic in man, pop up like mushrooms after a rain in newspapers and magazines, on television, and on the radio. But there are few, if any, guidelines for the nurse to help her inform her clients how these hazards can be avoided. A chemical is proven carcinogenic, but the public statement not only fails to recommend specifics as to how it may be avoided, but even fails to recommend avoiding it. We find pollution today in our air, water, food, and soil; and potential hazards even exist in noise and radiation. Research is continually being carried on in all these areas; but the nurse has the hard task of evaluating conflicting results, and an even harder one in deciding how she herself can be of most use.

A basic problem is the complexity of the subject. Pollutants

71

are numerous and varied. Many are difficult to detect. Their concentration varies geographically. Monitoring techniques are often inadequate. All this is one basic reason for the difficulty of research in environment pollution; another is that it is hard to determine precisely the degree of exposure to specific pollutants.[2-4]

Research is further complicated because pollutants that, according to tests, do not cause problems alone may be dangerous in combination with others; that is, synergistic relationships exist between pollutants. In a synergistic relationship, the danger from the two combined pollutants is greater than the sum of the individual dangers. For example, nonsmokers may inhale asbestos particles without much harm, since the particles are carried out of the lungs by the beating of cilia in the respiratory tract. Smoking, however, interferes with this natural cleansing process, and as a result smokers have a much greater chance of contracting asbestos-induced cancer. Sulphur dioxide also interferes with the function of the cilia, and when lung surfaces are exposed to airborne carcinogenic substances in combination with sulphur dioxide, the hazard of cancer is proportionately increased. It is not just the inhalation of asbestos which is significant; it is important whether or not one also smokes, and what pollutants exist in the food and water one may be ingesting. When we consider the myriad types of pollution and the millions of ways pollutants can interact, we begin to appreciate the difficulty of conducting research in the field, and the greater difficulty of identifying preventive measures. Odem observes that

> Pollutants are produced by natural ecosystems as well as by man's agricultural and industrial activity. However, nature by and large "treats" (that is, renders less harmful), recycles, or makes good use of her pollutants. In the past man has counted on nature to treat his pollution as well. As the twentieth century comes to a close the sheer volume and increasingly poisonous nature of man-made pollutants threatens the integrity of nature and the cultural development of man. There is no way to avoid pollution entirely . . . but there are many ways to curtail the amount and to reduce the harmful impacts.[4] We are now presented with some imperative questions. One is this: is our pollution inevitable in a technological society, or is it caused by carelessness, haste and greed?[5] It is not an exaggeration to say that the answer may also be the answer to the question of whether or not man will survive on the earth.[4]

AIR POLLUTION

Ehrlich tells us that, "Air pollution kills. Since it usually kills slowly and unobtrusively, however, the resulting deaths are not dramatically called to the attention of the public."[2] But many studies have been done, and plentiful statistical evidence exists to show that urban dwellers breathing polluted air experience more disease than dwellers in less polluted areas.[6,2] The effects are most severe on those already in a poor state of health; the aged, the infirm, the poor, and the young suffer most heavily.

One major pollutant is sulphur dioxide, coming mainly from electric plants and coal-burning factories. Not only does this in itself irritate the respiratory tract and damage the lungs; by reducing the action of cilia, our built-in cleansing agent, it enchances the potential health hazards of other pollutants. Another is carbon monoxide, whose primary source is automobile emissions. By combining with the hemoglobin of the red blood cells in place of oxygen, it produces a hypoxic state. In small amounts, it causes dizziness, headaches, and fatigue. It is especially dangerous to person suffering from heart disease, respiratory disease, or anemia.

VIGNETTE

Bolling, a 34-year-old computer operator, comes in to talk to the nurse about his "tension headaches." Bolling works for a large insurance firm in the metropolitan area of the city and he commutes daily from a suburb that is a drive of an hour and a half away. In describing his headaches, Bolling says they begin late in the afternoon and by the time he gets home he has an awful headache and feels really "worn out" and "tired."

When a client like Bolling tells the nurse that he has repeated headaches and fatigue, she should investigate the possibility that they are caused by an environmental pollutant. Headaches occurring in the car on the way home from work may not be the result of tension, but perhaps of the high levels of carbon monoxide built up on our streets by stop-and-go traffic.

The sulphur oxides have a synergistic relationship with many other environmental pollutants, since they interfere with the way the body protects itself from foreign particles. A worker in an area with high amounts of sulphur oxides, such as an urban industrial area, is recklessly multiplying the dangers of his environment by smoking. Smoking contributes further to pollution of the lungs, decreases further the action of the cilia, and can leave the body defenseless against microbes and infections.

Asbestos is a significant source of particulant air pollution, a type in which particulates, or minute pieces of substances, can damage the lungs and cause gastric cancer. Asbestos is very common in our daily lives. We use it to insulate our houses and to line our jackets, pot holders, and gloves. It appears in many electrical and building materials, as well as in the clutch plates and brake linings of our cars. We find it in substances as varied as rugs, yarns, artificial snow, cigarette filters, cardboard, mailbags, life jackets, asphalt, and clay used for pottery and sculpture.[7] Asbestos dust, particles so minute that they can neither be seen nor felt, is in such products as a result of normal wear and tear. Asbestos dust, of course, is freely produced in factories where asbestos is a material. This dust will cause certain cancers of the lungs, the pleura, and the peritoneum; the connection between asbestos and bronchial cancer is also well established.[8]

Those at greatest risk from this pollutant, obviously, are the workers in industries which produce products that contain asbestos. It would seem that the general population is not endangered, since the concentration of asbestos dust in the ordinary urban atmosphere is 10,000 times lower than the concentration considered acceptable for industrial workers.[8] But the specific environment often needs to be considered. Cases of cancer attributable to asbestos have appeared in populations living downwind of asbestos-processing factories, where the output of factory ventilators may be contaminating the air. Remember, these particles are so minute that they can't be seen or felt.

Bolling's example demonstrates the need for the nurse to do a thorough environmental health history for all her clients, including a discussion of potential health hazards at work. Symptoms may develop slowly. There may be a period of 20 to 40 years between the first exposure to asbestos and the development of cancer. Counseling the young adult, therefore, is particularly important. In trades such as building and shipbuilding, where asbestos substances are used and precautions in their use are less fully developed than in factories, workers may need special education. The nurse cannot over-stress the fact that smoking is particularly hazardous for people who work with asbestos.

Another significant health hazard is freon, the gas used in aerosol spray cans. These products surround us. We use aerosol sprays for dispensing cooking odors, cleaning ovens, polishing furniture, and grooming, and for countless other tasks in our daily living. Millions of tiny particles are given off in clouds from the nozzles of these spray cans, particles *smaller than red blood cells*. These are breathed into the lungs or infiltrate into other body tissues such as eyes or skin.

Contrary to its reputation of being inert, aerosol propellant gas, freon, is rapid-acting and a potent cardiac toxin. Youths who have inhaled it have died of ventricular tachyarrhythmias, acute heart failure, and asphyxia.[9] There is some evidence that the epidemic asthma deaths in England from 1960 to 1967 may have been caused by sensitization of the heart to cardiac arrhythmias by the fluorocarbons used to propel bronchodilator aerosols,[10] that is, by a medication spray sold over the counter. Hair spray may cloud contact lenses. Insect repellants with an oil base may cause lipoid pneumonia. The body has no way of defending itself against the tiny particles that make up the spray mist.[11] Countless examples could be given, and Dr. Bertram Carnow, head of Occupation and Environmental Medicine at the University of Illinois Medical School, states that any aerosol spray should be considered a potential hazard.[11]

Recently, concern has developed that the freon escaping from aerosol cans, as well as that from refrigerators, freezers, and car air conditioners, may even be affecting the ozone layer of the atmosphere, the layer around the earth which protects us from the ultraviolet rays of the sun. If it is destroyed, it cannot be replaced. If this happens, there would be a significant increase in the incidence of skin cancer, and it is possible that life itself on our planet might be threatened.

The nurse should counsel clients, particularly those at risk, such as young children, the elderly, and clients with respiratory and cardiac diseases, not to use any kind of aerosol sprays. Indeed, she would do well to inform all young adults of the potential danger of aerosol sprays, so that they can protect themselves from becoming dependent on these easy-to-use products. These products are so pervasive that she may not succeed; but she can try to persuade them. She could suggest an interesting family exercise: collecting together all aerosol spray products in the house, not merely those in bathrooms and closets, but also those in kitchen, laundry room, workshop, garage, and basement. This could lead to the discussion of substitutes, such as roll-on for spray-on-deodorant. Most people are surprised when they see to what extent this convenient but dangerous product has infiltrated our daily lives.

NOISE POLLUTION

Noise is another source of pollution. For the past 25 years it has been increasing at the rate of 1 decibel per year. It is impossible to establish an accurate measure of noise annoyance level since this differs widely from person to person. It is, however, possible to establish a noise danger level. Although this has been done, the U.S.A.F. Recommended Maximum Level of Sound is regularly exceeded by such common objects in our lives as an idling bus, a subway train, a food blender, an outboard motor, a power mower, a motorcycle, and music with amplifiers 4 to 6 feet away.[5]

Deafness is better correlated with frequencies than with overall intensities of sounds, since most noises in urban communities are complex and composed of sounds of many frequencies which vary in intensity. A sudden severe exposure to loud noise can cause deafness. Chronic, long-term exposure to critical noise levels in industry or the community can cause insidious hearing loss.[5] It was once thought that noise effected only injury to the eardrum, the inner ear, or the acoustic nerves, but it is now realized that the effects are more far-reaching.

Apparently, noise causes a narrowing of the arteries which affects the hearing mechanisms, and the noise levels which cause this contraction occur during both sleep and wakefulness. Sutterly and Donnelly observe that

> Not only do noise signals make the blood vessels contract, but the skin becomes pale, muscles constrict, and adrenalin is shot out into the bloodstream. This adrenalin output causes tension and nervousness. If chronic, it can elevate blood pressure.[5]

With the proliferation of noisy machines, man has perhaps over-adapted to them. We are so accustomed to noise that it is difficult for clients to consider it a source of pollution. The nurse, therefore, should do routine hearing assessments and offer various suggestions. Clients can consider noise pollution when buying kitchen appliances or yard equipment; they can turn off the television when they are not actually viewing; and they can plant shrubs to act as sound breaks if they live on heavily traveled streets. But the nurse should go beyond merely providing her clients with anticipatory guidance. She can take an active part in local planning, emphasizing the need for zoning and ordinances to decrease noise in town or city; and she can campaign for adequate acoustical standards in homes, apartments, hospitals, schools, and industrial buildings.

WATER POLLUTION

A cross section taken of 969 public water systems in the United States has yielded disturbing results:[5] 41 percent of these systems deliver water of inferior quality; 36 percent contain bacteria or chemicals exceeding safe limits; 79 percent are not inspected annually; and 9 percent are actually dangerous. Pollutants of water can be chemical, biological, or physiological. Although we have significantly reduced the transmission of waterborne diseases, with the growth of population and industry, vast amounts of chemical and other pollutants are continually being added to our public water supplies. Agriculture makes increasing use of pesticides, herbicides, and nitrates, many of which end up in water glasses on the dinner table. These are not only a threat to the streams, rivers, and lakes where we swim (or perhaps more accurately, where we used to swim); they also threaten our health.[12] In some communities, adequate water-treatment facilities are a real problem, and in some instances citizens have been warned to boil their drinking water. Sometimes certain comparatively simple methods can be taken to insure better water. The nurse can suggest a few home remedies,[13] but these hardly get to the heart of the matter. Citizens in general need to become more active in policing the safety of the water they drink, and the nurse can play an important and influential part in this campaign.[13]

As yet, exact knowledge is lacking as to the effect of various types of water pollution on health. There is some data to indicate that areas where the supply of water is naturally soft are marked by a higher incidence of heart disease than others. Since the hardness of water will vary considerably from community to community, the amount of sodium in the water will vary; but clients who have water softeners should know that cooking with the hot, or softened water, will significantly raise their amount of sodium intake, a potential danger in developing heart disease.[14,15] Lead in water pumped through lead piping also poses a significant health threat. If the nurse's clients use their own wells, and not a community water supply, they should have the water tested regularly to see if it contains the bacteria *Escherichia coli*, as well as to see whether or not it is contaminated by any heavy metals or other chemicals such as nitrates, salt, or pesticides.

CHEMICAL POLLUTION

Pesticides contaminate not only water, but also food. Studies done on agricultural workers in areas where pesticides were used report signs of neurological disturbances such as those found in myasthenic patients.[16] Because of poor living conditions and health hazards, the average life span of migrant farm workers is 45 years, as compared with the average expected life span of 70. Recently, in a factory producing a potent insecticide, severe neurological symptoms such as shakes and loss of memory appeared among the workers, as well as sterility and liver and brain damage. In that community, 55 percent of the air was contaminated by insecticide. The effect of chemicals, such as additive nitrates in our foods, is discussed in Chapter 3, Nutrition and the Young Adult.

The nurse can counsel her clients to thoroughly wash or scrub foodstuffs to remove traces of pesticides. She can encourage clients in a position to do so to grow their own vegetables in their backyards or on their rooftops. Growing plants contribute oxygen to the atmosphere and thus in themselves counteract pollution. In addition, the home gardener is free to abstain from the use of pesticides and chemical fertilizers. He can instead make his own compost pile and garden organically. Particularly among young adults, interest in this field is rapidly growing. A great deal of literature is available, and the nurse can offer encouragement and a bibliography to anyone fortunate enough to be in touch with the land.[17-19]

RADIATION HAZARD

Nuclear technology and the use of radiation in medicine, public health, agriculture, and industry is arousing concern about radiation pollution. Here again exact standards are difficult to establish. It is difficult to calculate how much radiation can be received without genetic or ill effects. However, we do know that the effects of radiation are cumulative. The nurse should alert her young adult clients to the danger of unnecessary exposure. For example, they can be told to keep an accurate record of all x-rays they receive, particularly routine dental checkups. Accidents or illness difficult to diagnose often involve a number of x-rays. Nowadays people move from one community to another with increasing frequency. If they brought their x-ray records with them, they would not run the risk of being subjected to repeated unnecessary x-rays in a new place. High-risk workers, such as dentists and dental assistants, should be reminded of the importance of protecting themselves and their patients; many people, for instance, do not know that they should wear lead-lined aprons whenever they receive dental x-rays.[20] These high-risk workers should also be reminded to make sure that their equipment is checked regularly.

Another source of radiation, often forgotten, is the sun. Avoiding excessive exposure to the sun is one of the safeguards against cancer. Young adults should be cautioned against the popular pasttime of sunbathing. Since the effects of solar exposure are cumulative, it may well not be until the middle years that skin cancer from this cause may develop in a young adult. Some research indicates that sun exposure may cause malignant melanoma, and excessive sunlight has also been shown to inhibit deoxyribonucleic acid (DNA), ribonucleic acid (RNA), and protein synthesis in human skin.[20,21] For protection, preparations such as sunscreen or sun lotion should be used. Aminobenzoic acid, which they contain, is one of the best protective agents, and after excessive sweating or swimming it should be reapplied.[21]

ENVIRONMENTAL HEALTH HAZARDS —
THE ROLE OF THE NURSE

The common symptoms in pollution of all types include fatigue, listlessness, sleepiness, and headache. If these are present in clients, the nurse should investigate potential health hazards in their environment.

Beyond providing anticipatory guidance, nurses are in an excellent position to make their influence felt in the community, particularly in the area of health teaching. How widely known, for instance, is the danger of the aerosol spray? Obtaining accurate and up-to-date information is not easy, for although there is much interest and activity in the field, research is complicated and difficult and results are often contradictory. The nurse can keep abreast of developments through television and popular magazines, as well as through professional literature. Prevention of pollution begins with an informed community, and the nurse has much to offer here.

There are today many groups deeply concerned with environmental quality, such as the Nature Conservancy, the Sierra Club, Friends of the Earth, and others. They are working actively to protect us against many dangers heretofore unrecognized. By example, the nurse can often help to enlist others in what may come to be recognized as our highest endeavor: the preservation of a safe environment.

BIBLIOGRAPHY

1   Murray, Ruth, and Judith Zentner: *Nursing Concepts for Health Promotion*, Prentice-Hall, Inc., Englewood Cliffs, N. J., 1975.

2* Ehrlich, Paul R., Ann H. Ehrlich, and John P. Holdren: *Human Ecology*, W. H. Freeman and Company, San Francisco, 1973.

3   Lave, Lester B., and E. P. Seskin: "Air Pollution and Human Health," *Science*, 169: 723–733, 1970.

4* Odum, Eugene P.: *Ecology*, 2d ed., Holt, Rinehart and Winston, Inc., New York, 1975.

5   Sutterley, Doris Cook, and Gloria Ferraro Donnelly: *Perspectives in Human Development: Nursing Throughout the Life Cycle*, J. B. Lippincott Company, Philadelphia, 1973.

6   Commoner, B.: *The Closing Circle: Nature, Man and Technology*, Alfred A. Knopf, Inc., New York, 1971.

7   Dohner, V. A., et al.: "Asbestos Exposure and Multiple Primary Tumors," *Am. Rev. Resp. Dis.*, vol. 2, 112: 181–199, 1975.

8   Barnes, R.: "Asbestos and Malignant Disease," *Med. J. Australia*, 2: 1107–1112, 1972.

9   Harris, W. S.: "Toxic Effects of Aerosol Propellants on the Heart," *Arch. Intern. Med.*, 131: 162–166, 1973.

10   "Flurocarbon Aerosol Propellants," *Lancet*, 1 (7915): 1073–1074, 1975.

11   Jaub, Samuel J.: "The Dangers of Aerosol Sprays," *Eye, Ear, Nose Throat Monthly*, 51: 347, 1972.

12   Yobs, Anne R.: "The Impact of Changing Pesticide Usage on the Medical Community," *J. Oklahoma State Med. Assoc.* 66: 360–362, 1973.

13* Harris, Robert H., Edward M. Brecher, and the Editors of Consumer Reports: "Is the Water Safe to Drink? Part 3: What You Can Do," *Consumer Reports*, 39 (8): 623–627, 1974.

14   Lewis, M.: "Softened Water," *J. Am. Med. Assoc.*, 228: 978, 1974.

15   McGarvey, J. F.: "Sodium Content of Water-Softened Water," *J. Am. Med. Assoc.*, 1258, 1974.

16   Drenth, H. J., et al.: Neuromuscular Function in Agricultural Workers Using Pesticides," *Arch. Environ. Health*, 25: 395–398, 1972.

17* Langer, Richard W.: *Grow It*, Saturday Review Press, New York, 1972.

18   Stout, Ruth: *How to Have a Green Thumb Without an Aching Back*, Cornerstone Library, Inc., New York, 1955.

19* Tyler, Hamilton: *Organic Gardening Without Poisons*, Van Nostrand Reinhold Company, New York, 1970.

20   Smith, N. J.: "The Hazard to the Dentist and His Staff from Dental Radiology," *Dental Practice Dental Record*, 22: 409–413, 1972.

21   Kammester, L. H.: "Sunlight, Skin Cancer, and Sunscreens," *J. Amer. Med. Assoc.* 232: 1373–1374, 1975.

22   Movslovitz, M., et al.: "Role of Sun Exposure in the Etiology of Malignant Melanoma: Epidemiologic Inference," *J. Nat. Cancer Inst.* 51: 777–779, 1973.

23* Ehrlich, Paul R., and Ann H. Ehrlich: *The End of Affluence*, Ballantine Books, Inc., New York, 1974.

*Starred items are of particular interest.

Living Sensibly # The Middle Adult

PART TWO

CHAPTER 6

Middle Adulthood– An Overview

In the middle years, all of us inevitably notice in ourselves the signs of physical aging. The nurse can help clients understand that although this is a natural process which can not be avoided or escaped, they do have a choice: They may refuse to admit it, they may fight it, and they may resort to useless cosmetics or dangerous drugs; or they may accept it, make the best of it, and age gracefully. In our American society an exaggerated importance is placed upon youth, which is after all only one stage of the full life development, and one which like every other has both strengths and weaknesses. The nurse can show clients the strengths of middle age, which lead on to the strengths of old age.

SENSORY CHANGES

The first physical signs of aging are often associated with changes in the sense organs. *Presbyopia*, or farsightedness, is extremely common in middle adults, even in those who have not previously had any vision problems. This can be easily corrected by eyeglasses that will be needed for reading or close work.

Other vision changes include decreased acuity, decreased sensitivity in the dark, and decreased peripheral vision, all the result of the cornea becoming less transparent and thus admitting less light. The latter two conditions may not allow for correction with glasses. Decreased peripheral vision could perhaps be compensated for by shifting the eyes more often and thus maintaining a wide field of vision. These changes have more dangerous implications than presbyopia since if decreased adaptation to the dark becomes significant, it may be necessary to limit driving to daylight hours. These changes are subtle and slow and therefore not easily detected. It is important that the middle adult be aware of their probability, and take steps to anticipate trouble before it arises. It is an excellent time to establish the habit of a routine eye examination every year.

Presbycusis, or impaired auditory acuity, is another common sensory change in middle age. First to be lost is usually the ability to hear the higher sound frequencies, such as a woman's voice or a bird's song. Unfortunately, people who are hard-of-hearing are often treated in our society with an impatience and discourtesy to which the visually impaired are not often subjected. The person with impaired hearing may have difficulty in taking part in conversation, especially in social groups. Deafness serves as an isolating factor in a way that blindness does not. A hearing aid is less common than eyeglasses and therefore more of a stigma; it is also a more blatant sign of aging, since people of all ages wear glasses but hearing aids are typically worn only by the old. The nurse can encourage clients to have routine auditory evaluations and to instill in clients the importance of this test as a part of a routine physical examination for middle adults.

MUSCULOSKELETAL CHANGES

After adult stature is reached, musculoskeletal integrity generally begins to decline. There is a decrease in bone density and mass. The middle adult starts to "shrink." Vertebral compression may occur with resulting backache; arthritic complaints commonly begin in middle age. Middle adults begin to "feel the weather in their bones" and notice soreness in joints. This is due in part to accumulated wear and tear on the joints and is aggravated by the presence of obesity.[1,2]

Muscle tone also gradually decreases, and muscle cells are replaced by adipose and connective tissue, resulting in a flabbier appearance and decreased strength. This decrease in muscle tone and muscle cells, however, does not necessarily affect endurance, only the strength and speed of the muscle reaction.

As long as the middle adult follows a routine exercise program that involves strenuous exercise, he or she may maintain endurance. Though a father may no longer beat his son at tennis, if he jogs routinely he may have more endurance than the son who takes time to jog only on weekends. A mother who does plenty of walking may have more endurance than her daughter who takes the car every time she goes to the corner drugstore.

CHANGES IN PHYSICAL APPEARANCE

We are all familiar with the term "middle-age spread." Weight gain is common in this period for two reasons: the metabolic rate decreases without a corresponding reduction in caloric consumption; and many adults lead more sedentary lives than before. Hair usually begins to turn gray. Women complain of thinning hair, men of baldness. The skin becomes dry and scaly. Decreased cutaneous fat results in less turgor and in sagging and wrinkles, sending flocks of men and women to doctors for cosmetic surgery. The overall balance of facial features alters; the face appears coarser or more bony and the nose more dominant.

American men and women spend billions of dollars each year on cosmetics in the hope that they can reverse these changes. Ignorant of the physiology of aging, they purchase hormone creams, cucumber juice, or queen bee extract "guaranteed" to preserve the youthful appearance which is so important in our youth-oriented society.

But it is quite possible for the middle adult to take advantage of these changes. When the pigment in the hair-producing cells disappears so that hair is white, this offers many an entirely new range of becoming colors to wear. Men and women may find they can now wear reds or blues. While hair color often changes and the skin's pink tint begins to yellow, eye color does not; the eyes become the dominant, exquisite feature of the aging portrait. To clients for whom appearance is important, the nurse can encourage middle adults to experience the harmony of the changes they are undergoing.

DECREASED BASAL ENERGY EXPENDITURE

In middle age, the basal, or resting, energy expenditure of the body begins to decrease, and less oxygen is utilized. As a result, there is a decrease in the amount of blood pumped by the heart and air expired by the lungs under resting conditions. There is a consequent decline in physical work capacity and energy. Thus people cut down on social activities. "We're getting old. We can't stay out late like we used to." They avoid picking up events in too rapid succession, so they can recuperate between them and enjoy them more thoroughly.

DECREASE IN FUNCTIONAL CAPACITIES OF ORGAN SYSTEMS

In aging, there is a reduction of the number of normally functioning cells, and due to this degeneration every physiological system becomes less efficient. For example, a decrease occurs in the amount of gastric juices secreted, which may lead to problems with "acid stomach" and belching.

Perhaps the most dramatic and far-reaching changes occur in the cardiovascular system. As a result of connective tissue replacement and calcium salt deposits, blood vessels become increasingly inelastic. The walls become thicker and the lumen smaller. Coronary artery disease, hypertension, myocardial infarction, cerebral vascular accidents, and peripheral vascular disease are some of the pathologies associated with the blood vessel changes of aging.

INCIDENCE OF DISEASE

Middle adults have a higher incidence of disease, especially chronic problems, than do young adults. These include the previously mentioned cardiovascular diseases as well as obesity, arthritis, deafness, eye problems, diseases of the female reproductive system, and depression. Cancer in the female and heart disease in the male are the leading causes of death in the middle adults.[3]

CANCER

What causes cancer? Many factors have been identified, ranging from jobs, food, worry, smoking, and air pollution to family background, chemicals, viruses, alcohol, and sex. All these factors and others play a part in causing different forms of the disease. An effort is now being made to identify people at greatest risk, whether because of family background, jobs, drugs, or life-styles, in order to improve preventive measures. But much work remains to be done.

Present studies do indicate that women with a family history of cancer run 6 to 9 times the risk of developing the disease than others do. Also, women whose menstrual cycles started early or who became mothers late seem to run increased risk here. Prostitutes, who have frequent sex with many partners, run a greater risk of cervical cancer than less sexually active women.[4]

Smoking increases the risk of lung cancer tenfold. No single known measure would lengthen the life or improve the health of the American population more than would eliminating cigarette smoking. Smoking not only increases the risk of cancer in and of itself, but also combines adversely with other factors, such as working where asbestos dust is inhaled or drinking excessively. We have conclusive proof that, with few exceptions, cancer of the lung is caused by smoking, usually cigarette smoking; this is therefore the one cancer which is preventable. It is tragic that this preventable cancer is increasing more rapidly than all others.[5]

While the causes of cancer are not clear, four areas are under current investigation. The first involves food and drink. Foods and food additives may contribute to cancer through complex chemical interactions that have only recently come under scrutiny. One example is the controversy over sodium nitrate and sodium nitrite. A high-fat diet seems to be linked with the risk of two of the most prevalent malignant diseases, cancer of the bowel and of the breast.[6] Also, a diet lacking fiber seems to be linked with colonic cancer.[7] Excess in alcohol seems to be related to cancers of the mouth, throat, esophagus, larynx, and liver.

The second field of investigation is drugs. One of the most disturbing links between drugs and cancer was discovered in 1971, when the daughters of women who took the synthetic estrogen diethylstilbestrol (DES) in early pregnancy were found to be susceptible to an often fatal vaginal cancer. Between 1969 and 1973, according to a study directed by Dr. Noel Weiss of the University of Washington, the incidence of uterine cancer increased at least 40 percent and as much as 150 percent in the middle-age women.[8] The study concluded that the drug estrogen, which is used to cure many of the discomforts of the menopause, probably was responsible for this dramatic increase. In another study,[9] the conclusion was that there is a high level of statistical significance to the hypothesis that estrogen causes uterine cancer. In this study, the disease was found to appear from 4 to 8 years after the women stopped taking the drug; generally the greatest risk was among those who took the largest doses over the longest periods. Estrogen can be a valuable drug, but should be used with prudence. Finally, the question remains unanswered as to whether or not the birth control pill influences the development of cancer. One study showed the existence of risk; three others failed to show any connection.[6]

The third area of investigation is radiation. Without question, x-rays and similar forms of radiation can cause leukemia and other forms of cancer if received in high doses. However, it was recently discovered that children who received radiation for tonsilitis, enlarged thymus glands, and other conditions during the 1940s and 1950s have an increased risk of thyroid cancers.

It is not clear at present how much risk exists from exposure to conventional diagnostic x-rays. Authorities disagree. Some say there is no evidence that 1 rad (standard unit of dosage) carries any risk. According to Lorne Houten of Roswell Park Memorial Institute, however, the amount of radiation from a single abdominal x-ray significantly increases the risk of leukemia.[6] One rad of radiation ages the cells it strikes by 1 year; thus a 50-year-old man who receives 10 rads has the susceptibility to nonlymphatic leukemia (a form of the disease that strikes adults) of a 60-year-old. Irradiation of men and women during their reproductive years, Houten believes, increases the likelihood that their offspring will develop leukemia. Below the age of 50, therefore, no one should undergo routine screening x-rays, including mammography to detect breast cancer (an exception, according to Houten, is the woman with a family history of breast cancer).

Woman under 35 whose family history shows no cancer should perhaps not have routine mammograms, or xeroradiography. The nurse should encourage clients to discuss this matter with their physicians. Whether repeated mammography can in itself increase the risk of developing breast cancer we do not know, but we do know that breast tissue is sensitive to the carcinogenic effects of radiation.

Ultraviolet radiation from the sun increases the risk of skin cancer. Evidence indicates mortality from skin cancer is 75 percent higher in the Southern states running from Louisiana to South Carolina than in the northern latitudes from Washington, D.C. to Minnesota.

The fourth area of investigation is the workplace. The list of substances that threaten Americans here is long and growing longer. Benzene increases the risk of leukemia in rubber workers. Inorganic arsenic contributes to a high incidence of lung cancer and lymphoma. Vinyl chloride is linked to liver cancer. For 80 years it has been known that benzidine, used in dye making, causes bladder cancer; the substance has been withdrawn in Great Britain and in the Soviet Union, yet it is still in widespread use in the United States.[6]

Concern exists not only for workers but also for their families and for persons living near plants that use hazardous substances. For example, people living in communities where there are copper-smelting facilities have a higher than expected average incidence of lung cancer.

Many occupational carcinogens do their work in combination with other noxious agents. The incidence of lung cancer among asbestos workers who smoked was 8 times what it was for smokers in other industries (and 92 times the incidence found in non-smokers).[6]

Why do we not know exactly what causes cancer? First, it is thought that cancer is not one disease involving a derangement in the life of the body's cells, but at least a hundred separate ones. Only by studying the epidemiology of cancer in humans on a vast scale can the factors of the disease be determined. Only then will we be able to identify persons at high risk.

Identifying cancer causes is difficult for two other reasons. First, a long latent period exists, sometimes 20 or even 35 years, between the first exposure to a carcinogenic substance and the appearance of a malignant disease. Also there is considerable disagreement about how much of a substance may trigger cancer. Second, it is controversial whether testing in animals is a reliable indicator of what a substance will do to man.

There is general agreement on the need for more research. There is also general agreement on the need for strict laws that would mandate testing of all new chemicals and drugs for toxicity and cancer-causing tendencies—testing before, not after, they are admitted into our environment.

Prevention begins with a thorough annual physical exam that includes a pelvic examination and Pap smear for women. An oral examination to detect cancer of the mouth and a rectal examination for cancer of the bowel should also be part of the physical examination. A chest x-ray for smokers is often given by some physicians.

Women should do the monthly self-breast exam. The nurse has a variety of good teaching materials to use when teaching the self-breast exam. However, a very important part that is often neglected by the nurse is a client return demonstration. If a client can successfully teach you and show you on herself the self-breast exam, the learning has been successful. Thus when teaching clients this very important preventive practice, it is important to allow for later evaluation. Women who have demonstrated that they can perform the self-breast exam accurately should be encouraged to teach other women — regardless of their age. Older adult women may have some negative feelings about touching their breasts, but this procedure is as important to someone who is 65 as it is to someone who is 45.

Adults, particularly young adults, should be encouraged to avoid excessive exposure to the sun. Thus sunscreens, hats, and long-sleeved shirts should be encouraged.

The role of the nurse is to assess the clients' risk of developing cancer; to suggest modification to reduce risk if necessary and possible; to teach women the importance of a regular monthly self-breast exam; and to teach all clients the seven warning signs of the disease:

1 Unusual bleeding or discharge
2 A lump or thickening in the breast or elsewhere
3 A sore that does not heal
4 A change in bowel or bladder habits
5 Indigestion or difficulty in swallowing
6 Hoarseness or cough
7 A change in a wart or mole

If any of these conditions persists for more than 2 weeks, it is essential to see a doctor. A lump or thickening in the breast or elsewhere should be reported to the doctor immediately.

The nurse can encourage and participate in cancer detection programs.

HEART DISEASE

The number one killer of all adults in this country is heart disease. One-fourth of all deaths from heart attack and one-sixth of all deaths from stroke occur under the age of 65.

The most common form of heart disease is *hypertension*, commonly known as high blood pressure; hypertension is called the "silent killer" because it often has no recognizable symptoms. An estimated 23 million Americans have hypertension, though 50 percent of them do not know it. Blacks have a higher rate of hypertension than whites and suffer a higher death rate from it.[10] That hypertension be identified and treated is very important so that it does not become a chronic disease since it is in itself a risk factor for other serious forms of heart and circulatory disease.

All adults should be encouraged to have their blood pressure taken frequently; they should know their own, write it down, and keep track of it. Taking blood pressure is of course part of the regular physical exam, but in some clinics it can be taken at any time. Fortunately, hypertension can be treated and controlled.

Though hypertension, with treatment, may cease to be a risk factor for heart disease, a number of other risk factors exist. Among them is smoking; studies have shown that heavy cigarette smokers have twice the risk of heart attacks that nonsmokers, former smokers, or cigar and pipe smokers do. A third risk factor for heart disease is a diet high in saturated fats and cholesterol. A fourth is overeating, which results in weight gain and obesity. A fifth is diabetes. And a sixth risk factor is lack of exercise, since exercise maintains muscle tone, stimulates blood circulation, and helps prevent weight gain. Inactive adults tend to experience more severe types of heart attack, have higher death rates due to heart attack, and run a greater risk of having heart attacks in the future than do active adults.

A family history of heart disease is another serious risk factor. Adults, and even children, whose blood relatives (especially parents and siblings) have had heart disease before the age of 60 have an increased chance for developing it themselves at a comparatively early age. This may occur for genetic reasons or because they have life-styles in common. A part of this risk factor is sex, race, and age. Women are likely to develop heart disease after menopause. Blacks are twice as likely to develop it as whites.[10] For all persons the incidence increases steadily with age.

A final risk factor is psychological and social stress. Persons described as overly ambitious, highly motivated, and constantly on the go, as well as those under great pressure at home or at work, appear more likely candidates than persons of more relaxed temperaments and life-styles.

Preventive measures begin with an annual checkup which includes the taking of blood pressure and lab studies for cholesterol. An EKG is recommended annually for all adults over 40. If clients smoke, the nurse should urge them to stop, or at least cut down. They should limit the amounts of saturated fats and cholesterol in their diets, and if they are overweight or obese, they should reduce. They should increase their exercise. Finally, as far as possible they should free themselves of stress and anxiety.

A good exercise program may be helpful, or perhaps learning how to meditate. Meditation is by no means confined to mystics. It is an excellent way of reducing tension, infinitely preferable to alcohol or other drugs, and may be easily learned. Basically, it involves sitting comfortably in a quiet place, freeing the mind of all worrying thoughts, and focusing attention on a certain object, a word, or a phrase.

Just as an exercise program should suit the tastes and circumstances of its user, so should the type of meditation, and there is a good deal of variation as to the kind individuals may find most helpful. Since some systems involve a considerable expenditure of money, some preliminary investigation is desirable. Any city phone book lists meditation societies (yoga, zen, transcendental), or the nurse can suggest that clients consult a minister, priest, or rabbi.

Lastly the nurse should use community resources such as smoking clinics, dietitians, and the local American Heart Association in providing clients with the resources and information they need in reducing the risk of heart disease.

DEVELOPMENTAL TASKS

During this period, successful middle adults experience some psychological changes as well as physiological ones. This can be a time of great change for the middle adult and to be able to anticipate the developmental tasks can be quite helpful.

Separating From Parents and Children by Becoming Independent

The middle adult, in Eda LeShan's words, sometimes feels "caught between his children and his parents."[11] Some feel guilty at making a decision that their parents do not approve of, particularly when they reflect that their parents are growing older and may not have much longer to live. Others are overanxious to please their children, and adolescent children may make excessive, unrealistic demands. Frequently, older children (young adults themselves) are not grateful for what seems to them to be overprotectiveness and may resent it bitterly. Nor should they be grateful, since they themselves are in the process of establishing their own independence. The parents must say, in effect, "We've done our best. Now it's up to you. We always love you, but now you must assume responsibility for your life and your decisions."

Toward the end of the middle adult period, as both the parents and the children grow older, their ages normally bring about new developments which the middle adults must be prepared to meet. Their children leave home to make their own lives. While this generally frees the parents from financial responsibility, it also robs them of their role as parents. Women may find more difficulty in coping with this change than men, since often the father's role was far less time-consuming and energy-consuming than the mother's, and men can compensate for the loss by deriving added satisfaction from their work.[12] The children marry and have children of their own. Some middle-aged couples experience difficulty if they expect to have the same relationship with the child that existed before he or she married, or if they expect the son-in-law or daughter-in-law to be "just like their own."[12] The nurse, who has seen many family adjustments, can tactfully hint that a grandmother who wants to carry on the family traditions her son knew (Christmas cookies, Easter eggs, whatever) must remember that the daughter-in-law has traditions from her family that she wants her children to enjoy, and that the interest in baseball that a father and daughter shared may not be one of the interests shared by that daughter with her new husband.

The loss of the children is exacerbated by our new social mobility. The continuity which existed when a son took over the family farm from his father no longer applies. Today, to an unprecedented extent, the children of blue-collar workers go to college and as a result have few tastes or interests in common with their parents. The farmer's son, for instance, gets a doctorate in biochemistry, marries, and settles down in a big city as a faculty member of a large university. The son of a maintenance man becomes a professional violinist who plays with a large metropolitan symphony. The second-generation families have moved far away from their parents; they have different occupations, different recreations, different friends, different interests, and different lifestyles. But family bonds remain. By anticipating these differences and dealing with them, parents and children can still maintain very important meaningful contact with each other.

In this period also the relationship of the middle adults to their own parents is likely to change, and they must be prepared to meet this change. For most middle adults, parents now are elderly, and this can present problems even more difficult and distressing than those involving children. The most successful way to deal with these problems is by facing them early—before they become so acute that they call for extreme means, which may result in great unhappiness, bitterness, and feelings of guilt.

While elderly parents are still in good health, self-reliant, and able to make decisions adapted to a variety of possible situations which may arise, middle-aged children should discuss future possibilities with them. If it has not occurred to them to do so, the nurse can suggest this type of assessment. It must be admitted that even in cases of careful planning, the role reversal in which a daughter becomes a mother to her mother, or a son a father to his father, can be a difficult one. To force elderly parents to leave their own home against their wishes—often this involves a recent widow or widower—is distressing for any sympathetic child and may produce a keen sense of guilt. But on the whole, difficulties are lessened if conditions are explored together by middle-aged children and elderly parents before a crisis arises.

Among the hazards listed by Bischof[13] which threaten good social and personal adjustments of the middle adult in terms of family life are opposition to a child's marriage, inability to establish a satisfactory relationship with a son-in-law or daughter-in-law, and providing care for an elderly parent. The nurse, who has seen how many clients cope with these events, can provide anticipatory guidance to middle adults "at risk" in these areas. But success will depend very largely on how successful they have been at achieving independence for themselves from their children and their parents.

Achieving Self-esteem Through Self-awareness Middle adults who do not use the middle years to deepen their sense of self-esteem often complain that life is growing boring and dull. Left to themselves, some middle adults allow their horizons to shrink, not expand; they recognize their failing powers and changes in appearance, they complain that life is over for them, and they sink into depression.

This is quite unnecessary. They have achieved, in most cases, a very fortunate position. The responsibilities of childbearing and child rearing are behind them, and they may have both economic security and time for self-development. They have freedom for experimentation: they can do what they "always wanted to do." It may be entering a new career, starting a business of their own, going back to school, taking the summer off, or touring the country. All of these offer opportunities for growth. Through these types of experiences they will learn more about themselves.

Few of us achieve self-awareness without pain. And one painful concomitant of this period is that the relationship between man and wife often changes, just as does that between middle adults and their children and middle adults and their parents. Bischof lists sexual adjustments, divorce, and remarriage as among the hazards at this time.[13] When a man and wife were in their twenties, they were raising their children, working hard for career or business advancement, and perhaps too occupied to give time or thought to self-awareness. Now with children gone and with decreasing job pressure, they are conscious of empty time; they look at each other and perhaps see the face of a stranger. The divorce rate is very high among middle adults, as are the rates of remarriage and suicide. It may be possible for the nurse to help by suggesting that this period need not result in a rift, but an opportunity to form a new and stronger relationship—a second coming together.

Learning more about one's self and discovering one's assets can involve periods of pain and joy. Developing or strengthening a love relationship or seeking a new career can help the middle adult increase his self-esteem through self-awareness. The nurse should encourage middle adults to expand their horizons and to use these years as a time to grow.

Reviewing One's Value System The middle adult needs to feel secure about the foundation on which values are based. Values change along with everything else, sometimes too rapidly to be judged during years that are filled with parenting or the pursuit of a career. Middle age allows time to go back and reexamine them. The usual result is that some values are discarded, others are retained, and confidence is enhanced for having taken stock.

Some middle adults, now freed from their parental roles, experiment with new social behaviors or activities that as parental-role models they were reluctant to do. This experimentation can take the form of examining the new trend of fathers becoming more involved in the process of childrearing.

The nurse should support clients and encourage them to look closely and carefully at their values, especially those established in adolescence and young adulthood. There is potential for growth in an examination of what to discard, what to alter, and what to hold as meaningful, and the nurse has a responsiblility to help the middle adult recognize that potential.

Preparing for the Future For the middle adult, the future means retirement and old age. Retirement is a complex issue with financial, social, and geographic implications. It needs to be prepared for early. This task involves anticipating and planning for the next stage of growth, older adulthood. Frequently such planning is based upon current abilities and interests.

It is important to give thought to developing new sources of enjoyment, since inevitably some current interests disappear as one ages. Because it is impossible to know which physical abilities will begin diminishing first, it is valuable to cultivate a variety of activities involving all of the senses: music for hearing, painting and reading for sight, knitting or carpentry for touch, cooking for taste, and flower or herb gardening for smell. Much of what is dreaded about old age can be minimized, and much of what is happily anticipated can be increased if the middle adult begins to prepare for retirement and old age early.

The nurse, in providing anticipatory guidance to the middle adult, should assess the growth in each of these developmental tasks. It is not necessary that the nurse personally belong to this age group; what may be lacking in firsthand experience can be compensated for by observation. The nurse can increase her expertise in this area through contacts with a wide range of clients.

BIBLIOGRAPHY

1* Smith, David W., and Edwin L. Bierman: *The Biologic Ages of Man from Conception Through Old Age*, W. B. Saunders Company, Philadelphia, 1973.

2 Simon, Anne W.: *The New Years: A Very Middle Age*, Alfred A. Knopf, Inc., New York, 1968.

3 *Statistical Bulletin*, Metropolitan Life (Source of Basic Data: Reports of Division of Vital Statistics, National Center for Health Statistics), New York, Sept. 1975.

4   Auerbach, Stuart: "Doctors Find All Kinds of Factors Leading to Cancers," *Chicago Tribune*, p. 20, April 15, 1976.

5   Ochsner, A.: "Cancer of the Lung—A Preventable Disease," J. Am. *Dietetic Assoc.*, 62: 249–252, 1973.

6*   Clark, M., et al.: "What Causes Cancer?" *Newsweek*, Jan. 26, 1976, pp. 62–67.

7   Hill, M. J.: "Bacteria and the Etiology of Colonic Cancer," *Cancer*, 34: 815-818.

8   Donald C. Smith et al.: "Association of Exogenous Estrogen and Endometrial Carcinoma," *New England Journal of Medicine*, **293**: 1164-1167, 1975.

9   Harry K. Ziel and William D. Finkle: "Increased Risk of Endometrial Carcinoma Among Users of Conjugated Estrogens," *New England Journal of Medicine*, **293**: 1167-1170, 1975.

10   "High Blood Pressure," Wisconsin Heart Association, January 1975.

11* LeShan, Eda: *The Wonderful Crisis of Middle Age*, David McKay Company, Inc., New York, 1973.

12* Hurlock, Elizabeth B.: *Developmental Physchology*, 4th. ed., McGraw-Hill Book Company, New York, 1975.

13* Bischof, L. J.: *Adult Psychology*, Harper & Publishers, Incorporated, New York, 1969.

*Starred items are of particular interest.

CHAPTER 7

Sensible Living: Exercise, Sleep, Special Problems

Just as sensible habits formed in young adulthood can lead to healthy, happy middle age, so sensible habits formed in middle age can retard aging and minimize its undesirable effects. Middle age means inevitable and natural changes, but the nurse can help clients deal with them realistically. Exercise and sleep will be discussed, as well as two special problems encountered in many clients, cigarette smoking and the abuse of alcohol.

EXERCISE AND ACTIVITY

From recent medical research we have evidence that premature aging is accelerated by inactivity. True, other factors are involved, such as heredity and diet, but a major factor seems to be physical stagnation due to lack of exercise.[1]

To some extent, this may result from the material values which Americans are often alleged to rate too highly. Middle age is generally the period in which earnings increase, and middle adults like to show off and be admired for what they can buy. If a man can afford a snow blower, he throws away his shovel. His wife prides herself on the number of machines in her home which do her work for her, while her mother perhaps and her grandmother certainly had to do the washing and sweeping with their own hands. Neither man nor woman may realize how inactive he or she is becoming. Both are "busy" all day long, aren't they?

Also, attempts at physical exercise may be laughed at. The man who decided to walk up the two flights to his office got tired of answering the question, "Why didn't you take the elevator?" The woman who mowed her lawn with an old-fashioned hand mower had to defend her husband against the charge of stinginess. "Why doesn't your husband buy you a power mower?"

But perhaps the greatest problem for the middle adult who wants to increase exercise is overcoming a present state of physical unfitness. As we have said, obesity is a very common and serious problem in this period. This is also the time when a chronic illness may develop, and for various reasons, clients may physically be very unfit. The nurse cannot overemphasize that two steps should precede any attempt to increase exercise: assessment of present level of activity and assessment of physical fitness. Only then should a program of exercise be developed—and that gradually. Suddenly taxing the body with spurts of exercise can endanger health and indeed life itself.

The Administration on Aging has published a useful pamphlet planned to provide physical conditioning through a careful well-planned exercise program to improve the health of the cardiovascular system.[2] It contains a simple pre-exercise Walk Test and Walk-Jog Tests to determine present condition and exercise tolerance. If at any time during the Walk Test the clients experience any trembling, nausea, extreme breathlessness, pounding in the head, or pain in the chest, they should stop *immediately*. These are signs of reaching their present level of exercise tolerance. Each client should start the keep-fit programs at this individual tolerance level, and if the symptoms persist beyond the point of temporary discomfort, consult a physician.

Exercisers should start out slowly, very slowly, and step up the tempo and number of repetitions very gradually; this method will keep stiffness and soreness to a minimum. Some stiffness can be expected during the first few days and is no excuse to stop; it's a sign that the exercises are badly needed, and it will soon disappear.

While exercise should be tailored to an individual's physical condition, it should also be adapted to life-style and individual taste. Walking is an excellent suggestion for the nurse to offer, for it is very adaptable. You can take a walk around the neighborhod after dinner to see what is going on, who has the best crop of dandelions, who is moving out or in, or what's on sale at the grocery or drugstore. If you want a reason, you can walk to the library, or to pick up the newspaper. You can take a side trip and thus extend your range. All sorts of possibilities open up, and, very happily, many experimenters quickly become addicted to this beneficial habit.

Senator William Proxmire, a crusader for walking, insists that a great sense of well-being comes with the ability to walk long distances without tiring.

> "You feel stronger and you are. You sleep better because you're physically tired, feel far less tense and nervous. The next time you feel angry, frustrated, tense or irritable, instead of taking aspirin, a tranquilizer, or a shot of whiskey, take a walk.
>
> You'll find that a walk is a far greater benefit to your nerves and your emotions than any artificial calmer-downer."[3]

He could have added that walking costs nothing.

Walking is also adaptable in that it can be done alone or with a companion. A loner might enjoy it, or might enjoy working out at home to music or while watching television. But the gregarious person would enjoy group activity more, and the nurse should have suggestions here. Some possibilities for locating physical fitness groups include the YMCA and YWCA, service clubs, parks and recreation departments, and local college courses. It is to be remembered that self-discipline in any area usually is easier when undertaken with others.

The influence of Far Eastern cultures is spreading rapidly in the field of physical fitness. Young and not-so-young persons are accepting the challenges of karate, belly dancing, and the like, finding them refreshing mentally as well as physically. A particularly appropriate discipline for middle adults is Tai Chi Chuan, a series of slow-paced circular movements that flow into each other to form a graceful, stately dance. It has been called a "near perfect" exercise for older people because it imposes no strain, yet demands correct posture, balance, breathing, and concentration.[4] In advanced forms it provides an effective method of self-defense utilizing an opponent's movements and requiring little strength of one's own. But for all, its rewards include increased strength and vitality and a tranquil mind.

For some middle adults it is difficult to find time for any "additional" exercise. Very easy to do, once you start, is adaptation of everyday movements that turns chores and daily routines into beneficial exercises. Any motion can be used to bring a variety of muscles into play. For example, walking can be done occasionally on tiptoe, with knees bent; while you are sitting, toes can be flexed and clenched and knees flexed and extended. A daily walk to the bank, by a gradual increase of pace, can become a daily jog. If you drive to work, you can park a few blocks away and then walk; if you go by bus, you can take it a few blocks from your home and get off in the evening as far away as you like. If you park your car at a far corner of a shopping center, you can get in a good walk to the store. This sort of thing can become an entertaining game.

What is the best type of exercise for the middle adult? There are several requirements: it should increase the efficiency of the heart and lungs; and it should be continuous, rhythmic, and for a period long enough to stress the circulatory system. Recommended forms include brisk walking, jogging, swimming, bicycling, and skipping rope. As you progress, action should be gradually increased until it can be sustained hard and long enough to keep the pulse rate above 130 for several minutes and increase the body temperature gradually to the point of perspiration.[4]

The late Dr. Paul Dudley White, the eminent heart surgeon, stressed the importance of the use of the leg muscles in walking, bicycling, and the like, in order to maintain proper circulation and to prevent cardiovascular disease.

He wrote,

Studies have shown that when a person is walking about 30% of the circulation of the blood is carried on by the leg muscles and the remaining portion by the heart. Vigorous leg muscle exercise is probably one of the best methods known to keep the veins clear and to prevent the formation of blood clots.[4]

Usually, persons over 40 should engage in sports that emphasize skill and coordination rather than speed, strength, and endurance; they should avoid those sports that require sudden starts and stops, or put sudden strain on weak parts of the body, such as the back and legs. Persons over 50 should be even more cautious, particularly when starting a new activity. To look at the other side of the coin, persons over 50 who have been athletic all their lives should be counseled to cut down on the amount and vigor of their exercise, especially if breathlessness, rapid pulse, or pounding heart persists for more than 10 minutes after exertion. Other warning signs of overexertion are dizziness, tightness or pain in the chest, nausea, and loss of muscle control.

Gradual increase and *maintenance* are therefore key words in a health-exercise program for the middle adult. Dr. Cooper says in *The New Aerobics*, "Exercise is the medicine that keeps countless people alive. But like all medicine it must be taken according to prescription."[1] The nurse should point out that before exercising a warming-up period of stretching and rotating muscles is very important; after exercise a cooling-off period is also necessary, during which activity gradually decreases. Exercisers should stop before they become exhausted. And above all, both the nurse and doctor who know the clients' physical condition should be aware of any program undertaken. Too often men and women begin strenuous exercise programs which get them into trouble—trouble which would be avoided if they had first consulted a professional. Finally, the nurse, familiar with clients' life-styles, can be creative in suggesting what activities will appeal to them and supportive as the client begins to include them in his daily life.

SLEEP

For the middle adult, sleep patterns slowly change from those of the young adult. There are two particular changes: middle adults spend less time in deep sleep and they need less sleep overall (see Chapter 2). These normal changes may give rise to a perceived problem of insomnia. Middle adults following the same sleep schedule they used when younger may have difficulty falling asleep or may wake up very early; this is not insomnia, as they may think, but an expression of the body's need for less sleep.

In *Better Than Ever*, Dr. Joyce Brothers suggests this procedure for a week:

> Take the clock out of the bedroom and make sure that windows are heavily curtained so that the morning light won't awaken you; then go to bed when you feel sleepy and get up when you wake up. Make a note of the hours you have slept. Over a week, you will have a good idea of your true sleep needs and they will probably be less than you thought.[5]

It is important that the sleep middle adults get is of good quality, since with aging it will become less in quantity. Some middle adults may feel tired during the middle of the day, and the nurse should encourage them to take a nap if it is possible. If it is not, they might take one in the late afternoon or evening when they get home from work.

USE OF MEDICATIONS

Middle adulthood is for many a period of a good deal of stress and anxiety. By and large, it is the period in our lives when all sorts of responsibilities weigh most heavily upon us. Therefore many people may find great difficulty in falling asleep at night. Fear of a sleepless night, with resulting fatigue and inefficiency the next day, will only increase the anxiety which prevents sleep. Many people, indeed far too many, take medication to help them sleep, some prescription drugs, some over-the-counter drugs; and it is easy for the middle adult to become dependent on these.

It can safely be said that both hypnotics and tranquilizers interfere with the quality of sleep.

> In general, major tranquilizers decrease the waking period. However, major tranquilizers with strong extrapyramidal side effects, such as peperazine, phenothiazine, thiothizene, haloperidol, and molidone, also decrease State IV sleep,"[6]

Low dosages may decrease it, high dosages may increase it. Not only stage IV, but also stage I (light sleep) was observed to shorten. As for minor tranquilizers and hypnotics, they had a marked effect on REM periods, decreasing their length as well as burst and single REM activity. It is to be remembered that a night's sleep is not a continuous plateau, but a series of cycles, and that for good quality sleep each stage must run its course. Whatever interferes with the cycles, then, decreases this all-important quality of sleep.

Over-the-counter medications for sleep are often a waste of money, frequently having no effect. Moreover, they can be actually dangerous when taken in combination with other over-the-counter medications. For instance, when sleeping aids such as Nytol, Sominex, and Sleep Aids are taken in combination with alcohol, allergy or cold remedies, cough syrups, cough and cold remedies, antihistamines, or tranquilizers, these can enhance the depressive effects of the sleep medications and cause drowsiness, mental dullness, and the lack of ability to concentrate the next day. When taken in combination with other antidepressants, such as Elavil or Vivactyle, they can cause dry mouth, blurred vision, or constipation, and can seriously aggravate glaucoma, if that condition exists.[7] So it is important that the nurse inform clients of the implications of sleep medications, especially in combination.

According to Dr. Charles C. Edwards, former Commissioner of the Food and Drug Administration, over-the-counter preparations sold to induce sleep or ease tensions are nearly worthless. A placebo, about 35 percent of the time, would also produce improvement in the symptoms. And under controlled conditions, when sleep is needed or tensions just need to be relaxed, placebos actually do much better than nonprescription drugs, curing up to 70 percent of the symptoms.[8] The nurse should try to educate clients to free themselves from drug dependence and use other methods, such as a glass of warm milk, to secure sleep of good quality.

Since the deep refreshing sleep of adolescence and young adulthood is significantly diminished in this period, middle adults may feel, wrongly, that they "haven't slept a wink." They probably slept; but the sleep was most likely the lighter stages, not only less refreshing than deep sleep but sometimes almost indistinguishable from wakefulness and punctuated with periods of it. The wakeful spells and the lighter sleep may easily deceive clients into thinking they need medication unless the nurse provides anticipatory guidance to help them adapt to the normal changes of their period of life.

Knowing these changes in sleep patterns may help middle adults not only to accept them but even to enjoy them. To wake early and lie in bed watching the sky lighten is a better way to start the day than sleeping through the alarm, rushing over preparations, finding fault with the family, and getting oneself and everybody else off to a bad start.

Two special problems will be discussed here. The nurse will encounter them in many clients, and though they have generally started before this period, it is now they can become particularly serious in relation to physiological changes. The first problem is cigarette smoking.

SMOKING

According to the U.S. Department of Agriculture, the average per capita consumption of cigarettes in the 1970s for persons over the age of 18 has been over 4000 cigarettes per person. About 75 percent of the male and 50 percent of the female population smoke. More people smoke in cities than in the country. The habit is usually formed first at about age 12; it is estimated that about 1 million teenagers become smokers annually. For both adults and teenagers, more smokers occur among those with less formal education and in the low socioeconomic brackets. But for both men and women, the larger number of cigarettes smoked occurs among those with high educational achievement and high incomes.[9]

Studies indicate that adolescents are more likely to smoke if their parents do, and older brothers and sisters, cousins, aunts, and uncles also have an important influence. Adolescents are likely to imitate any admired adult—teacher, minister, doctor, or nurse—who smokes. Some smoke as a way of experimenting with adult life, others to show rebellion against authority.

Sometimes peers urge the younger smoker to start. If he or she is in a group where it is the thing to do, it will be hard for the adolescent to stand out. Another strong factor is advertising, which implies that smoking is modern and desirable and will win the smoker both male and female friends. Once the habit begins, it continues, and it may later become closely associated with pleasant events, such as social gatherings or the first cup of coffee in the morning. Smoking seems to relieve tension to such a point that the smoker becomes very anxious if it is not possible to smoke. Although smoking is not addicting in the physiological sense, psychological dependence can develop.

EFFECTS OF SMOKING
Basically, smoking shortens life.

> According to Linus Pauling, the eminent physicist and Nobel laureate, an individual aged 50 who has smoked more than a pack of cigarettes a day since the age of 21 has an 8½-year shorter life expectancy than an individual the same age who has never smoked. He has calculated on the basis of statistics that for every cigarette one smokes, one's life is shortened by 14.4 minutes.[10]

From studies currently being done, we are acquiring more specific information on the effects of smoking. According to the American Medical Association, just ten puffs of a cigarette increases resistance in the air pathways of the lungs, and this choked-up condition persists for an hour after each smoke.[1] When one smokes, the carbon monoxide from the smoke rapidly enters the bloodstream, combines with the hemoglobin in the red blood cells, and affects their oxygen-carrying capacity. This decrease in the ability to carry oxygen affects the body's ability to carry oxygen from the lungs to the muscles. The nicotine in the cigarette increases the requirement of the heart for oxygen, while the carbon monoxide inhibits the blood from supplying it. These two conflicting factors put a strain on the heart which may ultimately result in coronary heart disease. This is particularly true if the smoker is also obese, hypertensive, inactive, or has high serum cholesterol.

In habitual smokers, the lung capacity shrinks and the membranes of the air passages thicken and become less efficient in gas exchange. The lungs lose their elasticity, and both inhaling and exhaling become extremely difficult, a significant factor in emphysema.

When one smokes, the millions of *cilia*, tiny hair-like moving structures that act as a broom and sweep out the windpipe and the bronchial tubes, become paralyzed. Thus tiny foreign particles such as dust, pollen, and soot can accumulate in the linings of the bronchial tubes. Allowing cancer-causing or cancer-promoting substances to remain in contact with the tar that also accumulates promotes the development of cancer. Cancer often begins in the bronchial tubes and spreads into the lungs. Approximately 90 percent of all cases of lung cancer originate in people who smoke cigarettes. A rare disease 50 years ago, this is now a primary cause of death from cancer.[9]

Cancer of the larynx, esophagus, mouth, pharnyx, and cheek has also been associated with smoking. Pipe smokers seem to be at risk for developing cancer of the lip. Other studies have linked smoking to cancer of the bladder, pancreas, and kidney.

There is strong evidence to indicate that smoking mothers have a significantly greater number of unsuccessful pregnancies due to stillbirth and neonatal death. Smoking has also been implicated in spontaneous abortions (miscarriages).[11]

In general, nonsmokers are in better health than smokers. A National Health Survey showed that between the ages of 45 and 64, men who smoked were disabled by illness at a rate 28 percent higher than were men who did not.[9] Smokers become winded more easily and they develop "smoker's cough" in their attempt to rid the lungs of the foreign substances which the cilia normally handle.

Smoking affects not only the smokers themselves but also nonsmokers. Infants and children, who cannot protect themselves, as well as the elderly, can be subjected to risk through the ignorance or self-centeredness of smokers. The rights of nonsmokers are only just beginning to receive recognition.

PROCESS OF SMOKING

Whether or not a smoker will develop a smoking-related disease depends on several variables: average number of cigarettes consumed daily; length of time smoking has gone on; and depth of inhalation. There is a direct correlation between decreased life expectancy and the number of cigarettes smoked and the depth of cigarette smoke inhalation.

Stopping smoking increases life expectancy at once. Despite all the damage of smoking, the body is able to reverse many of the effects once it is stopped. The cilia resume their function and clean the lungs, lung capacity improves; the smoker's cough disappears. All the effects on the heart may not be reversed, but since circulation is increased it is subjected to less strain.

To stop smoking involves several factors. It is never easy to break a habit, and to break this one seems to present particular difficulties. Smokers often have built-up pleasant associations with a certain brand. Smoking is often done while socializing with others. Certain activities at certain times of day seem to lose their savor without the accompaniment of a cigarette—say, relaxing after dinner at the end of a hard day's work. The actual physical manipulation of the cigarette, striking a match and lighting up, seems important to some people, giving them "something to do with their hands." None of these factors can be ignored.

HOW TO QUIT SMOKING

VIGNETTE
Esther is a 55-year-old widow who smokes a pack of cigarettes a day. Having her blood pressure taken (she is slightly hypertensive), she discusses with the nurse her frustration in trying to stop smoking. "Every time I really get down to it, either I put on a lot of weight or I get angry and irritable at everyone I see. I'm in the clothing business, and I can't afford to do either of those. What should I do?"

If clients want to succeed, they must first have a real desire to stop—a desire based on the sound knowledge that to continue to smoke will virtually guarantee ill health and perhaps an early death, and may also produce ill effects on the health of others they care for.

Next the nurse should help the client assess the patterns and factors of smoking (see Chapter 16). Then the client is ready to begin.

The client should be told to choose a day, one fairly free from stress, to start. Cut down on those cigarettes which you have identified as wanting the least. In a few days, go on to eliminate the ones you feel you wanted more. After a short period you will be ready to cut out the ones you want the most.

During this period avoid the things that make you want to smoke. If possible, avoid other smokers. If you enjoy smoking with other people, do not take a cigarette unless you leave the crowd to light up—this will make you question how much you want to do it. If you want something to do with your hands, handle a key or pencil or some other small object. If you smoke to relax, try some other method: exercise, meditation, eating (but only if you are underweight). If you want the lift smoking seems to give you, try the diet brands of carbonated colas, which may do as well. If you find yourself smoking automatically, try to figure out what triggered your doing so. If it was a cup of coffee, switch to tea. If it was opening your purse and seeing matches, stop carrying matches.

There are some anti-smoking drugs which may help you satisfy your craving, since they contain lobeline, which is similar in action to nicotine. Lobeline is available in over-the-counter preparations, but it is essential that you discuss the matter first with a physician, since some people cannot tolerate it, and for others it is not effective.[12]

HOW TO LOWER YOUR INTAKE OF CIGARETTE SMOKE

Some people have seriously tried to quit smoking and failed. For them, the nurse can make the following suggestions to lessen the hazard:

1. Choose a cigarette with less tar and nicotine. Free cards are available from the Federal Trade Commission rating the tar and nicotine contents of the major brands of cigarettes sold in the United States so that you can determine the amounts in the brand you use.

2. Don't smoke your cigarette all the way down. The greatest intake of tar and nicotine occurs in the last few puffs. The tobacco itself acts as a filter, and the first half of the cigarette yields only 40% of the total.

3. Take fewer draws on each cigarette. You will be actually cutting down if you take fewer puffs, even if you can't stop.

4. Reduce your inhaling. It is the smoke that enters the lungs that does the most damage. Pipe and cigar smokers are less likely to have smoking-related diseases than cigarette smokers, because they usually inhale less.

5. Smoke fewer cigarettes each day. Try to change your habit pattern by smoking only one cigarette at a time, and by postponing a cigarette as often as you can. If you promise yourself one later, it is often easier not to take one now.[13]

The nurse's role is to help clients who smoke, pointing out the hazards involved not only to themselves but also to others, and urging them first to assess their smoking habits and then to reduce smoking or stop altogether. This may be very difficult for nurses who are smokers themselves. Many health care people today, however, are beginning to realize the implications of this habit for themselves; they recognize that it is detrimental to their own health and to the rapport between them and their clients. As the seriousness and prevalence of this problem grows, groups and smoking clinics which may be a source of help are beginning to appear in many communities. These may be found at a local hospital, school, or other community service organization. The nurse should be aware of those that exist to which clients may be referred.

DRUG USE AND ABUSE

During the middle years the nurse can help clients to accept the changes and stresses of these years and make the best of them by their own efforts, without dependence on drugs. Of course, many clients will be taking medications individually prescribed for them by their physicians. We have already discussed tranquilizers and hypnotics in connection with sleep. However, the greatest drug problem in our culture today is that of alcohol.

ALCOHOL
Alcohol, by medical definition, is a drug; it affects the central nervous system and causes other physiological changes. Popularly, however, it is not thought of as a drug, for it is sold without a prescription, and legally so.

It is important to distinguish between the person who drinks alcohol and the alcoholic. For many people, alcohol is simply an amenity of life.

Says Dr. Chafetz, director of the National Institute on Alcohol Abuse and Alcoholism,

> Among cultures which use alcoholic beverages, but are little troubled by alcohol problems, the general tendency is to sip alcohol slowly, consume it with good food, and partake of alcohol in the company of others in relaxed comfortable surroundings. Drinking is taken for granted, and given no special significance, and no positive value is attributed to prowess in amounts consumed. Moreover, intoxication is abhorred.[13]

But Americans often drink liquor as they live life—rapidly and tensely—and this has led to some frightening statistics. There are roughly 9 million citizens with serious drinking problems in the United States. One out of every ten American workers is an alcoholic or has a serious drinking problem. Fewer than 10 percent of all citizens who have drinking problems receive any medical treatment.[14] Of the 9 million alcoholics, about 2 million are women; in the past 5 years the percentage of women in Alcoholics Anonymous has risen from 25 to 40 percent. There has been a recent increase in drinking among teenagers, and alcoholism now exists in that age group, which was previously thought impossible, since it was assumed that years of drinking were necessary to cause the condition.

At those two indigenous American institutions, the cocktail party and the commuter bar, drinking is usually done standing; the alcoholic beverage is gulped down rapidly with the barest minimum of food; and the general aim is to "get high" as quickly as possible. Even more significant is the fact that this pattern is condoned; it is frequently all right to drink just to get drunk. There are geographical concentrations of heavy drinking in our country today, one being Washington, D.C., where per capita consumption of alcohol is the highest in the nation.[14]

Perhaps some users of alcohol would not become abusers of it if they knew, and applied to themselves and their habits, some simple facts with which the nurse is in a position to furnish clients.

The effects of alcohol occur very quickly. As a mug of beer or a cocktail is consumed, 20 percent of it is absorbed instantly into the bloodstream through the walls of the stomach or small intestine. The gastrointestinal tract processes the remaining 80 percent at a very rapid rate. The bloodstream carries the alcohol directly to the brain.[9]

Thus only seconds after alcohol is ingested, it appears in all the organs, tissues, and secretions of the body. How quickly it goes to work on the brain depends on the interaction of several factors:

1   Rate of consumption. It takes most people about an hour to burn less than an ounce of alcohol. Drinking at a faster rate will produce some degree of intoxication.

2   Quantity of food in the stomach. Food slows down the rate of absorption of alcohol into the bloodstream. Drinking on an empty stomach causes the alcohol to reach the brain faster and so causes a faster response.

3   Kind of alcohol. Distilled spirits are absorbed into the bloodstream faster than wine or beer. The latter are less concentrated, have small amounts of nonalcoholic substances which are removed during distillation, and therefore have a slower absorption rate.

4   Additional mixers. Water dilutes alcohol and slows the rate of absorption. Carbonated mixers speed it up.

5   Body weight. Alcohol is distributed rapidly and uniformly throughout the circulatory system. A small person who is drinking the same liquor at the same rate as a large person will have higher concentration of alcohol at every point in his bloodstream because he does not have as much blood or tissue to dilute the alcohol.

6   Emotional condition. During periods of anxiety, stress, or fatigue, the chances are alcohol will go to work faster than under comfortable and relaxed circumstances.

7   Body chemistry. There are apparently some differences in individual body chemistry that affect the rate of absorption. Even when all other conditions are the same, alcohol can have a stronger impact on one person than another.[9]

THE ALCOHOLIC

The Skid Row derelict is for most of us the stereotype of the alcoholic, yet he represents only 3 to 5 percent of the alcoholic population.[9] The majority of alcoholics hold jobs, at least marginally. Many heads of families, home owners, professionals, and top executives are alcoholics. It was formerly held that only people inadequate and emotionally vulnerable would become alcoholics. This is a mistake. All types of personalities occur among alcoholics, and they are to be found in all social strata and in every possible occupation.

The line between heavy drinker and alcoholic is not clear-cut. Dr. E. Jellinek divides the development of alcoholism into four phases: pre-alcoholic, prodromal, crucial, and chronic. These do not necessarily always occur in the same order, nor does every alcoholic always exhibit every symptom.

> Alcoholism may occasionally develop on the basis of heavy socio-occupational drinking without the presence of marked personality problems. Individuals whose drinking "rewards" them with relief of their anxieties, tensions, and so on, tend to proceed from occasional to constant relief drinking. Whether heavy drinking starts on a psychogenic or a sociogenic basis, sooner or later it leads to an increase in alcohol tolerance. This necessitates the consumption of increased amounts of alcoholic drink in order to achieve the desired effect. This initial pre-alcoholic symptomatic phase leads to the prodromal phase with the onset of so-called alcoholic blackouts.[15]

During the prodromal phase, there is increasing dependence on alcohol, and drinking becomes surreptitious. Driving under the influence of alcohol may occur repeatedly. Drinkers feel an urgent need for the first drink, but also guilt at taking it. They may find it impossible to discuss their problem. Memory blackouts increase.

Loss of control marks the crucial stage. Drinkers cannot stop when others do. They may not go so far as actual drunkenness or uncontrollable vomiting, but they do not seem to know beforehand how any particular drinking occasion may end. They are torn between reasons for drinking and attempts at resistance, remorse, and futile good resolutions. They lose interest in their work, which is likely to involve them in money troubles. They avoid their friends and family. They lose interest in food, and as a result of neglect of proper food intake they may develop vitamin and protein deficiencies that can result in physical deterioration.

The main characteristic of the final, chronic phase is the "bender" —periods of prolonged alcoholic intoxication. Fortunately, most alcoholics never reach this stage—fortunately, for it is marked by physical and mental damage and moral deterioration. At this phase drinking is an obsession, the be-all and end-all of the drinker's life. This is the end of the road.[15]

The view was formerly widely held that alcoholics had to go all the way, reach rock bottom, lose jobs and money, alienate friends and family, and in desperation admit defeat before being willing to accept treatment with the chance of recovery. This view is wrong. All that is necessary is an honest desire for help, and this may occur at any point. Nonetheless, the way back on this road is long and hard.

Abstinence does not automatically guarantee the cure of the disease; yet it is highly important if for no other reason than that it provides reassurance to the family of the drinker, who have often been so painfully disappointed in the past. It is the view of Alcoholism Anonymous that alcoholics need to recognize that they are allergic to alcohol and must therefore avoid it. Some new evidence exists, however, that some alcoholics may be able later to resume some type of controlled drinking.[16]

Who is at risk for developing alcoholism? One group consists of professionals under great stress, such as doctors, lawyers, engineers, and people in business. But the true answer is anyone at all. Alcoholism in the family may predispose children to the disease, though a physiological cause or genetic link has not been conclusively established. There does appear to be good evidence that children are greatly influenced by their parents' drinking habits. The first drink, on an average, occurs at the age of 13 or 14, usually at home. Most teenagers who use alcohol do so with their parents' permission.

ALCOHOLISM

The importance of alcoholism as a disease is obvious. Since symptoms vary and very few sufferers are treated, it is important that the nurse be able to identify it. As is true in many diseases, the earlier the identification and diagnosis, the better the prognosis in general, and the nurse often sees incipient sufferers in the early stages. Theoretically, the long drawn-out period over which the disease develops provides ample time for preventive and early therapeutic measures; actually, however, too often these are not taken because of delay in diagnosis. Many alcoholics or pre-alcoholics enter and leave the health care system without ever being identified. The primary health care nurse is in an excellent position to identify alcoholism early, but this can be done only by sharpening of diagnostic skills and familiarity with the physical and behavioral signs associated with problem drinking.

J. L. Mueller lists five components to describe the role of the nurse as counselor in this field: contact, concern, communication, confrontation, and community.[17] Contact, as we have pointed out, means more than just being in the same room; it means the nurse's identification of the problem. The nurse must feel true concern—concern deep, sincere, and genuine. This cannot be faked; if it is, it will only rouse hostility. Concern must lead to communication. A difficulty arises here, for many drinkers are too defensive to admit their problems. The nurse can perhaps give factual information about the progression and danger signs of pathological drinking, possibly using diabetes or some other disease as a parallel, and thereby lead the drinker to look at the situation realistically and talk openly and frankly about it. The fourth point, confrontation, is risky and must be used skillfully and sincerely. It may sometimes be necessary to point out discrepancies between what the drinker says and what is actually the case. If this is done ineptly, it may precipitate a crisis with the result that the nurse can be of no more use to a person who badly needs help.

The community approach, finally, needs emphasis. A marked feature of alcoholism is that the sufferer, in most cases, brings troubles to others, primarily family members, and that these others may also need help. Successful treatment of the individual sometimes involves a combination of methods, such as hospital care, drugs, psychotherapy, and Alcoholics Anonymous. Alcoholics Anonymous, though perhaps the best known, is by no means the only organization which can help both the alcoholic and the alcoholic's family. There are many such in every community: church groups, mental health services, and the like. The nurse should be informed as to those which do exist. In a position of trust, with the advantage of a long-term relationship with the client and familiarity with the family, the nurse is well equipped to help and support them all.

Over 68 million Americans drink alcohol in some form, though fortunately it is only a small proportion of them who reach the extreme stage of becoming alcoholics. The nurse, however, has a responsibility not only to those clients who do, but to others whose health and safety may be affected by drinking.

A recent study has shown a relationship between cancer at various sites and the use of alcohol.[18] Generally, the more alcohol consumed, the greater the chance for developing certain types of cancer. For instance, heavy drinkers were 10 times more susceptible to oral cancer than moderate ones, all other factors being equal. Consumption of whiskey rather than wine or beer, it has been found, is more often linked to the development of cancer. This type of information should be passed on to clients.

Industrial accidents are another field for the primary health care nurse. Alcoholics contribute to a high rate of accidents on and off the job. The developing alcoholic under 40 years of age experiences 7 times as many on-the-job accidents as the fully developed alcoholic over 40.[19] A good practical rule for the nurse is that for the first accident for any worker, a check should be made on mechanical and environmental factors; for the second, a check should be made on the human factor, through the use of group consultation; for the third, perhaps a referral to a doctor, psychiatrist, or social worker is required.

Finally, the nurse has a basic responsibility to contribute to public education in the view of alcoholism as a disease. Today we are just beginning to realize that the place for a "drunk" is the hospital, not the jail. We still need to know a great deal more about this disease, including its causes and the most effective types of treatment. The nurse should be active in supporting programs that develop new techniques of prevention, treatment, and rehabilitation; that train professionals in their use; and that contribute to public enlightenment.

BIBLIOGRAPHY

1*   Cooper, Kenneth H.: *The New Aerobics*, Bantam Books, Inc., New York, 1970.
2*   *Adult Physical Fitness*, Superintendent of Documents, Consumer Information, Public Documents Distribution Center, Pueblo, Colo. 81009.
3*   Beverly, E. Virginia: "The Mechanics of Putting Those Little-Used Muscles in Motion," *Geriatrics*, 31 (1): 132-134, 1976.
4*   Beverly, E. Virginia: "An Assortment of Fitness Programs for the Unconditioned Retiree," *Geriatrics*, 31 (2): 122-131, 1976.
5   Brothers, Joyce: *Better Than Ever*, Simon and Schuster, New York, 1975.
6   Itil, Turan M.: "The Effects of Minor and Major Tranquilizers on Digital Computer Sleep Prints," in Uros J. Jovanovic (ed.), *The Nature of Sleep*, Gustav Fisher Verlag, Stuttgart, Germany, 1973.
7*   Silverman, Harold, Steve Grenard, and Gilbert I. Simon: *Med-File Drug Interaction System*, Med-File, Inc., Sarasota, Fla., 1976.
8   Mark, Norman: "Calm Down At Your Own Risk," *Today's Health*, Mar. 1974, pp. 16-19.
9*   Mayer, Jean: *Health*, D. Van Nostrand Company, Inc., Princeton, N.J.
10   Ochsner, A.: "The Health Menace of Tabacco," *AM. Scientist*, 59: 246-252.
11   Sabak-Sharpee, G. J.: "Is Your Sex Life Going Up in Smoke?" *Today's Health*, Aug. 1974, pp. 50-53.
12   "Smoking—What You Need to Know," Public Health Service Publication No. 1786, U.S. Department of Health, Education, and Welfare, National Clearinghouse for Smoking and Health, Rockville, Md.
13   Blakeslee, Alton and Brian Sullivan: "Teenage Drinking Is New Concern For Parents," *Capital Times Newspaper*, Madison, Wis., Mar. 25, 1976.
14   Shearer, Lloyd: "Parade Magazine," Wisconsin State Journal, Jan. 4, 1976.
15* Glatt, M. M.: "Why and How People Become Alcoholics," *Nursing Times*, 71:723-725, 1976.

16   Glatt, M. M.: "A Complex Interdisciplinary Disorder," *Nursing Times*, 71:680–682, 1975.

17*   Mueller, J. L.: "The Role of the Nurse in Counseling the Alcoholic," *J. Psychiat. Nursing*, 12:26–32, 1974.

18   Seixas, F. A.: "Alcohol, a Carcinogen?" *Cancer*, 25:62-65, 1975.

19   Nicholson, Richard E.: "Of Hooch and Hazards—Alcoholism and Accidents in Industry," *Occupational Health Nursing*, 22:10-12, 1974.

20*   Proxmire, William: *You Can Do It!*, Simon and Schuster, Inc., New York, 1973.

21*   Sloan, E. A.: *The New Complete Book of Bicycling*, Trident Press, Division of Simon & Schuster, Inc., New York, 1974.

22*   Sussman, A., and R. Goode: *The Magic of Walking*, Simon & Schuster, Inc., New York, 1967.

23*   deVries, H. A.: *Vigor Regained: A Simple, Proven Home Program for Restoring Fitness and Vitality*, Prentice-Hall, Inc., Englewood Cliffs, N. J. 1974.

*Starred items are of particular interest.

CHAPTER 8

Diet and Dieting

Rich foods—real whipped cream, best creamery butter, filet mignon smothered in sauteed onions, French fries—tend to make an increasing appearance on the tables of middle adults, whose increased income may now allow them to treat themselves and their guests. Eating in a restaurant may become a weekly affair instead of occurring only on Mother's Day. As sugars and fats increase in the diet, so too may bodily weight. Overweight and obesity are by no means limited to the middle years, but they are common enough then to give rise to the familiar term "middle-age spread."

Middle adults who put on weight probably do not know some established facts about this period of life. According to Williams, for each decade after the age of 25, caloric intake should be reduced by approximately 7.5 percent.[1] The reason is that during the middle years, metabolic activity decreases by about 5 percent; therefore the reduced basal energy requirements, caused by losses in functioning protoplasms and often by reduction in physical activity, are satisfied by fewer calories.

Other changes at this time may lead to certain complaints common in middle adults, particularly heartburn and constipation. Digestive glands secrete fewer gastric juices, often with the result of acid stomach and belching. Also, many middle adults acquire dentures and find chewing more difficult, especially of such excellent roughage foods as lettuce and celery. Constipation then becomes a problem. The nurse can provide anticipatory guidance at this time and help clients deal with these problems while they are merely incipient and therefore easily manageable.

MIDDLE ADULT DIET

In general, the only modification of the young adult diet necessary for the middle adult is a reduction in calories. In some cases, however, a chronic disease may appear and a specific therapeutic diet may be necessary. Diabetes and hypertension often occur at this time, for instance, and they require changes in diet.

Many middle adults, dismayed at the appearance of some of the physical changes of the middle years, think that vitamin and mineral supplements can retard the aging process or reverse some of the signs of aging. Unless prescribed by a doctor, commercial vitamins and minerals are not necessary. The nurse can expose the illusion that swallowing a capsule will stop hair from turning gray, increase sexual prowess, and bring back the bounding energy of youth, and can help clients to recognize that aging is a natural process.

NUTRITION AND DISEASE

Nutrition and diet have been suggested to be factors that influence certain diseases. Epidemiologic studies in human populations have implicated high levels of fat or a lack of fiber in the diet in the causation of breast and colon cancer. Differences in diet may bring about differences in intestinal microflora which have been associated with variations in the incidence of cancer of the large bowel. Colon-rectal cancer is a major cause of cancer death, second only to lung cancer in the United States.

Fiber is the dietary component which in recent years has received attention for its role in the etiology of cancer of the large bowel. The relationship between fiber content in the diet and colon cancer is unclear. However, several mechanisms have been suggested to explain how dietary fiber may reduce the incidence of colon cancer. Fiber decreases intestinal transit time, thereby reducing the duration of exposure of fecal carcinogens. Fiber also may exert a solvent-like effect in that it dilutes potential carcinogens by its bulking effect and ability to bind water, sterols, bile acids, and fats. Finally, fiber influences bile salt metabolism, thereby reducing the formation of potential carcinogens from bile salts.

More studies are needed to elucidate the mechanism by which nutrition and diet can influence carcinogenesis and to document associations between dietary practices and cancer. It is, however, premature to make specific dietary recommendations at present to minimize the risk of cancer, other than maintenance of desirable body weight.

According to the Framingham studies, there is a correlation between high serum cholesterol in the blood and heart disease (see Chapter 3). Much research is currently being done in the area of diet and heart disease. Middle adults would do well to restrict the amount of saturated fats in their diet, particularly since the normal American diet is high in saturated fat, which contributes greatly to obesity.

OBESITY

It is estimated that between 40 and 80 million Americans are obese. The number varies according to the criteria used. Since many people think of malnutrition as the result of eating too little, it may be a surprise to know that obesity is the commonest form of malnutrition in our affluent society. Broadly defined, obesity is a bodily condition of excessive, generalized deposits and storage of fats. The term "overweight" can be applied to being over-heavy without regard to fatness; thus a weight lifter could be overweight, but not obese.

We do not have good data on the prevalence of obesity for the population as a whole. According to insurance data, half the number of American men between the ages of 30 and 39 are at least 10 percent overweight and a quarter at least 20 percent overweight. The heaviest incidence is in the age bracket between 50 and 59; here 60 percent are more than 10 percent overweight and a third at least 20 percent overweight.[2]

If one uses height and weight charts as a criteria, 20 percent over the ideal weight is medically defined as obese, and 10 percent as overweight. There is, however, much current controversy over the desirability of height and weight charts as a measurement tool. The populations used to determine these charts are not necessarily typical, and such important aspects as body type and body frame are often not taken into account. Physicians and nutritionists are now beginning to rely less on charts and more on judgment—indeed on the client's own judgment. A man or woman is encouraged to look at himself or herself naked in a mirror; if she looks fat to herself, or if he looks fat to himself, well, then—he or she *is* fat.

Another useful test is the pinch test, which determines whether the density of skin pinched at various body points is greater or less than ½ inch. Still another test, perhaps most accurate of all, is the skin-fold measurement. With the use of external calipers, skin-fold measurements are taken in certain body areas. The measurement is compared with a scale to determine the degree of obesity. The triceps skin-fold, taken halfway between shoulder and elbow, is highly reliable. Other sites are the subscapular, abdominal, hip, pectoral, and calf areas, and accuracy is increased if several measurements are taken;[3] but the triceps site is probably the easiest and most representative. "While techniques such as densimetric, hydrometric, and whole-body potassium measurement, may be more precise, skin-fold measurement appears to be a more than adequately sensitive measure of obesity.[4]

OBESITY AS A RISK FACTOR

Obesity is a factor in diabetes and in cardiovascular and hypertensive diseases, as well as in a condition like arthritis, where it can cause a problem with mobility. The best treatment is prevention. In most cases the nurse is able to give this warning to a young adult. An obese middle adult carries increased risk, for at this time chronic diseases may appear; obesity may contribute to their presence and may also aggravate some of their symptoms.

It has been found that in the United States obesity is much more prevalent in the lower socioeconomic class than in the middle and upper classes. At present, explanations advanced for this finding are entirely conjectural.[5]

Obesity is particularly likely to make its appearance at certain periods. One of these, for both men and women, is the time when the body reaches its mature size and weight and the bones cease to grow. If food consumption then continues at much the same level as during the period of growth, the unused nutrients are stored as fat. Actually, after the age of 20, the muscle-to-fat ratio of the body changes; muscle tissue is reduced and is replaced with fat. Suppose a man at age 20 weighs 160 pounds and that approximately 12 percent of his weight is fat. At 55, if he has the same weight, 24 percent of it will be fat. Now suppose he gains 20 pounds during those 35 years; an even larger percent of his body weight will be fat, perhaps approximately a third.

There are two particular risk periods for women. Pregnancy is an event that may precipitate a large weight gain, particularly with the first baby, though the risk appears to be less with subsequent births. The age of the mother at the first pregnancy also affects the extent of risk. Only about 11 percent of pregnant teenagers become obese, but by the age of 35 the risk has increased until four out of ten first-time mothers do so.

The second risk period for women is menopause. Women in general tend to gain weight when menstruation stops, a gain which may be due to hormonal changes or to decreasing activity or perhaps to depression. A parallel pattern seems to exist in men, where a slow increase in weight seems to accelerate at about the age of 40. The primary cause for this is reduced activity.

TYPES OF OBESITY

According to Kemp, there are four types of obesity.[6] The first begins in childhood and continues up to about the age of 15. Obesity of this type is a real problem since weight reduction is much more difficult to achieve with children than with responsible adults. The second type has its onset between the ages of 15 and 25. This variety is less common, and when it occurs in males, it is usually due to less activity, more beer-drinking, and marriage. In this period, women seem more concerned than men with their looks and weight, and generally stay slim. The third type, however, is restricted to women, since it occurs during pregnancy; one-third of all obese females become so in relation to pregnancy. We have no evidence that hormones are at fault here; the cause is more probably the myth that the prospective mother should "eat for two." (See Chapter 3, on diet during pregnancy.)

The final type of obesity has its onset in the middle years, after the age of 35. In a study by Kemp, nearly two-thirds of the men became obese in their middle years as opposed to less than one-fourth of the women. The obese women had become so earlier, in childhood or pregnancy. Weight gain in the middle years is usually ascribed to too many calories and too little exercise. Throughout all these risk periods, the nurse can provide anticipatory guidance, always emphasizing *prevention*. It is easier to keep pounds off than to take them off.

CAUSES OF OBESITY

There are many factors which contribute to the condition of obesity. The following three factors can cause obesity, but they are only three of many identified factors of obesity.

Hereditary Factors There appears to be no significant relationship between birth weight and obesity. However, one study found that the child who is overweight at 6 months tends to be overweight at

5 years. Among the parents studied, when both were of normal weight, 8 percent of the children were obese; if one parent was obese, so were 40 percent of the children; and if both were, so were 80 percent of the children.[7] Withers suggests there is some evidence for genetic implications of obesity.[8] In a study of adopted children, their weights correlated with those of their natural, not their adoptive, parents. However, while genes may increase susceptibility to obesity, this is only one of many factors which predispose an individual to becoming obese.

Fat Cell Development Factor   The nutritional experiences of the infant can effect a permanent change in the number of fat cells.[9] According to Harper, infant feeding, intrauterine experience, and genetic factors all contribute to determining the number of fat cells,[10] which act as storage tanks. It has been found that the fat cells of the obese were both larger and more numerous than those of normal-weight persons. While the implications of this finding are still being explored, it is known that dieting can reduce the size of fat cells, but not the number. Approximately 80 percent of individuals overweight as children are also overweight as adults.[10] We do not yet know whether a child's diet can be modified so as to control or reduce the number of fat cells, whether the number is genetically determined, or whether it is influenced by the mother's diet. This factor, however, does seem to help explain why some adults carry on a life-long struggle against obesity.

Behavioral Factors   A good deal of study is now being done on the eating behavior of obese persons compared with that of persons of normal weight. Eating behavior is seen as a joint function of internal and external cues. Rapid eating, taking fewer meals per day, and lower activity have all been identified as significant factors for obesity. Some other contributing factors are conditioned or developmental inactivity and compulsive overeating. Using the knowledge of some of these factors that cause obesity, the nurse can answer the client's questions about why he or she may be obese.

CONTROL OF OBESITY
The average overweight person goes on 1.5 diets per year, and between the ages of 21 and 50, makes more than fifteen major attempts to lose weight.[4] Americans spend at least 100 million dollars a year on weight-reducing plans. It would be simplistic, to say the least, to state that obesity results from overeating, but without question the obese ingest more food than they need. The reasons

for this overconsumption, however, are very complex, and the nurse should guard against trying to fit all clients into one pattern. Gradually, as various comparative studies are being carried out, some sound evidence is being generated. According to one study, obese subjects ate less if they had to exert extra effort in the preparation of the food, while normal subjects ate the same amount regardless of whether or not they had worked hard in its preparation.[11] According to another, infrequent meals were associated with a tendency toward obesity.[12] It has also been found that fullness of the stomach does not affect the appetite of the obese; that they are more concerned with the taste of food than are normal weight persons; and that they eat more rapidly and eat more at a given time.

Dr. Stanley Schachter of Columbia University has studied how and when overweight and normal-weight people eat.[2] Research has shown the following:

1 Overeaters are much more likely to eat when food is in plain view and when it is in ready-to-eat form than when it has to be found and prepared.
2 Overeaters tend to eat only those foods which have special appeal to them and therefore, rather than "eating everything in sight," they have a few special weaknesses.
3 Overeaters tend to eat more when they do not know exactly how much they have eaten, but they eat carefully when they do know how much they are eating.
4 Overeaters are actually less likely to eat than people of normal weight when they become upset.

Psychological problems associated with obesity include loneliness, embarrassment caused by a lack of kindness toward the obese, depression, and a lack of interesting things to do, to mention only a few. Desperation, the companion of obesity, poses almost as serious a threat to well-being as do the risks of illness.

These data have been utilized in a behavioral approach to weight reduction by Stuart and Davis in *Slim Chance in a Fat World* (Condensed Edition). This book describes effective management of overweight by emphasizing situational and nutritional control and points out the importance of exercise.

Situational Control "Research has shown that what people eat, when they eat it, where they eat it, and how much of it they eat are all under what has been called 'situational control.' "[2] Eating behavior, then, is not under the control of the person himself, but it is under the control of the people with whom he lives and the places in which he carries out his life. Some of these controls are out in the open and others are hidden. Examples of these controls are TV commercials and women's magazines which sell cakes and cookies and other fattening foods. Have you ever seen a commercial for cauliflower? Other controls include the husband who brings his wife candy as a treat and the idea that a good host must always serve food.

Based on the current data about the behaviors of overeaters and the need to provide situational control, clients, according to Stuart and Davis, should be encouraged to keep food out of sight, buy nonfattening foods, eat in one room only, always shop with a list, do their shopping after they have eaten, measure all their portions of food, use smaller plates, train others to help them curb their eating (praise is needed, not punishment), and take steps to avoid loneliness, depression, anger, and fatigue. When people are very tired, they tend to try to obtain energy by eating. Clients should try to get enough sleep to keep them going comfortably.

Nutritional Control Learning to control the situation is only one part of successful weight control. Overweight individuals need to know what and how much they should eat. A complete dietary assessment is the place to begin (see Chapter 16).

Caloric allowances should be calculated (refer to *Slim Chance in a Fat World*, by Stuart and Davis, p. 40) to allow for a weight loss of 1 pound per week. People who lose more than 1 pound per week are more likely to regain this lost weight quickly.

Before beginning a reducing diet, clients should obtain a complete health assessment. Next, there are four essentials for a sensible good reducing diet. It should (1) be adequate in all nutrients and low only in calories; (2) comprise a variety of foods; (3) be adapted as closely as possible to the user's tastes and habits; and (4) provide for gradual retraining in eating patterns so that these patterns may become lifelong, allowing for suitable additions as they become possible.

Americans want to get rich quick and lose weight overnight. The former is difficult, the latter impossible. The nurse must warn clients against the plethora of crash diets widely publicized to cater to this demand (Air Force diet, Dr. Atkins's diet, Dr. Stillman's diet, kelp and B^6 diet, cider vinegar, and lecithin) and emphasize that a sensible diet is essential. Control of obesity is a long-term thing, and the diet is something to live with for the rest of your life. Otherwise you will simply be like the man who found it so easy to give up smoking he had already done it ten times.

The diet, as well as being sensible, must take the individual into account. Leveille and Romsos found that in some cases confining oneself to three meals a day might actually encourage obesity; as long as the day's intake of calories is watched, how they are taken is a matter of choice, and some people find nibbling helpful.[13] There are some general useful hints, however. Food should be kept out of sight as much as possible. Dieters who eat in restaurants can order clear broth rather than cream soup, choose broiled meat rather than fried, and nibble raw carrot and celery sticks to fill in the time waiting for the order to arrive instead of gorging themselves on hot buttered rolls.[14]

Exercise   Very large amounts of exercise are not necessary for weight control. But by moderately increasing the amount of exercise while dieting, people are able to burn off extra calories. Increasing exercise can be difficult for some adults who think it is "modern" to avoid exercise. There is also the myth that exercise increases one's appetite. Actually, the opposite is true. Moderate exercise serves to regulate appetite. Adults have greater appetites when they remain inactive than when they take moderate amounts of exercise.

Clients should be encouraged to try to increase their exercise to consume 500 calories per day. To do this, clients should increase their exercise using light, moderate, and heavy exercise activities. The following table is helpful in determining the amount of exercise an adult is receiving:

TABLE 9-1

Light exercise 4 cal/min	Moderate exercise 7 cal/min	Heavy exercise 10 cal/min
Dancing (slow step)	Badminton (singles)	Calisthenics (vigorous)
Gardening (light)	Cycling (9.5 mi/hr)	Climbing stairs (up and down)
Golf	Dancing (fast step)	Cycling (12 mi/hr)
Table tennis	Gardening (heavy)	Handball, paddleball, squash
Volleyball	Stationary cycling	Jogging
Walking	(moderately)	Skipping rope (quickly)
	Swimming (30 yd/min)	Stationary cycling and jogging
	Tennis (singles)	Swimming (40 yd/min)
	Walking (4.5 mi/hr)	

Exercising with a partner is helpful for most people. A client should select an exercise that fits into his style of living and place of living. Thus exercise like playing tennis, when it requires traveling miles to get to a court, really does not fit well into an individual's life. Exercise should be built into the client's day. It should become a part of the individual's life. Clients should be encouraged to pay themselves off or treat themselves when they have increased the exercise in their lives. A new dress, a size smaller, can do wonders.

Many dieters find support and help in joining with others. The two best known groups in this field are Weight Watchers and TOPS, both of which pursue a very sensible approach to dieting. Day hospital programs, directed weight control, and behavior-therapy group programs have also proved effective.[15-17]

In a problem of such national magnitude, nurses have a challenging opportunity to be of great use. They can not only dispel illusions and disperse facts; they are in an excellent position to support and encourage their clients.

BIBLIOGRAPHY

1* Williams, Sue R.: *Nutrition and Diet Therapy*, The C. V. Mosby Company, St. Louis, 1970.
2* Stuart, Richard B., and Barbara Davis: *Slim Chance in a Fat World*, condensed edition, Research Press Company, Champaign, Ill., 1972.
3 Sloan, A. W., et al.: "A Trial of the Ponderax Stronfold Caliper," *South African Med. Soc.*, 47:125-127, 1973.
4* Stuart, Richard B., and Barbara Davis: *Slim Chance in a Fat World*, Research Press Company, Champaign, Ill., 1972.
5 Mayer, Jean: *Health*, D. Van Nostrand Company, Inc., New York, 1974.
6 Kemp, R.: "The Over-All Picture of Obesity," *Practitioner*, 209:654-660, 1972.
7 Shukla, A., et al.: "Infantile Overnutrition in the First Year of Life: A Field Study in Dudley, Worcestershire," *Brit. Med. J.*, 4:507-515, 1972.
8 Withers, R. F. J.: "Problems in the Genetics of Obesity," *Eugenics Rev.* 58:81-84, 1964.
9 Knittle, J. L.: "Obesity in Childhood: A Problem in Adipose Tissue Cellular Development," *J. Pediat.*, 81:1048-1059, 1972.
10 Harper, P.: "Psychosomatic Medicine and Weight Disorders," *Practitioner*, 209:244-250, 1972.
11 Singh, D., et al.: "Role of Past Experience in Food-Motivated Behavior of Obese Humans," *J. Comp. Physiol. Psychol.*, 86:503-508, 1974.
12 Bray, G. A.: "To Nibble or Gorge?" *J. Clin. Invest.*, 51:537-541, 1972.
13 Leveille, Gilbert A., and Dale R. Romsos: "Meal Eating and Obesity," *Nursing Digest*, 4:18-20, 1976.
14 "Tips for Successful Weight Reduction and Remaining Slim," The Madison District Dietetic Association, 1975.
15 Westlake, R. J., et al.: "A Day Hospital Program for Treating Obesity," *Hospital Commun. Psychiat.*, 25:609-611, 1974.
16 Harris, M. B., et al.: "Self-Directed Weight Control Through Eating and Exercise," *Behavioral Res. Ther.*, 11:523-529, 1973.
17 Levitz, Leonard S.: "Behavior Therapy in Treating Obesity," *J. Amer. Dietetic Assoc.*, 62:22-26, 1973.

18   Crow, R. A., et al.: "Experimental Studies of Obesity," *Nursing Times,* 70:103–105, 1974.

19* Deutsch, Ronald M.: *The Family Guide to Better Food and Better Health,* Bantam Books, Inc., New York, 1973.

20   *How To Feed Your Family and Keep Them Fit and Happy . . . No Matter What,* Betty Crocker. Golden Press, New York, 1967.

21* *Eat and Stay Slim,* Better Homes & Gardens Books, Des Moines, 1968.

22* U.S. Supt. of Documents, *Calorie Counter.*

23* *Food and Your Weight,* Home and Garden Bulletin No. 74; *Nutrition Value of Foods,* Home and Garden Bulletin No. 72.

24* Mayer, Jean: *Overweight Courses, Cost and Control,* Spectrum Books, Prentice-Hall, Inc., Englewood Cliffs, N.J., 1968.

*Starred items are of particular interest.

CHAPTER 9

The Sexually Active Middle Adult

Most middle-aged Americans are victimized by a sexual stereotype that is culturally induced and perpetuated by commercialism. In our Western society, body beauty and physique tend to be equated with sexual desire and potency. Generally, it is acceptable to be chronologically old if one looks young, and to be sexually active if one looks attractive. Conversely, the aging body may be considered by some to be repulsive or even obscene. The advertising media has played a major role in perpetuating this myth. Models are generally either "beauties" or "uglies." The uglies promote paper towels and drain cleaners; the beauties promote cigarettes, liquor, cosmetics, and new cars. The beauties are generally slim, sleek, impeccably groomed and garbed, and almost always young. Many ads imply that the person who chooses brand A is discriminating in taste, successful in business, cultured, refined, and a tiger in the bedroom. Bombarded daily with these messages, it is little wonder that the middle-aged adult with thickening midriff, partial dentures, thinning hair, and sagging breasts may discount the possibility of offering continuing sexual attractiveness to a "significant other." Is loss of libido inevitable or circumstantial for those in the middle years? A review of the research on the physiological effects of aging and reported changes in interest and involvement in sexual activity will provide the nurse with important information to help her work with middle-aged clients.

One of the most enlightening reports about middle-aged sexuality comes from Duke University's longitudinal studies on aging. Pfeiffer and Davis obtained information about the sexual behavior of 502 whites aged 45 to 69 years, mainly of middle and upper socioeconomic status.[1] They concluded that the most significant contributing factor to current sexual functioning, including interest in, frequency, and enjoyment of sexual relations, was previous sexual experience. Income, social class, objective physical function rating, and expectation of future life satisfaction were positively correlated with current sexual function. For women, intact marriages and being employed were also positively correlated with present sexual function. Furthermore, the enjoyment of sexual relationships in younger years, rather than the frequency, seems to be of particular importance in determining a middle-aged woman's current interest in and frequency of sexual intercourse.

Hunt's study of sexual behavior in the 1970s concludes that the greatest sexual liberation has occurred among married people. Coital frequency has increased and is more egalitarian as to which partner initiates and which refuses. (The highest increase was found in those aged 56 to 60, who reported a frequency of once a week, as compared with once every other week reported by the Kinsey sample.) There is increased freedom to vary sexual positions and behaviors with large increases in mouth-breast activity, manual manipulation of the penis, and oral techniques. Over 70 percent of those who found married sex very pleasant have a close relationship; very few have good sex and a poor marital relationship. This seems to indicate a reciprocal relationship between the two variables that is worth emphasizing.[2]

COMMON SEXUAL PATTERNS FOR MARRIED
MIDDLE-AGED ADULTS

Assuming that the desired family size has been achieved, procreation for the middle adult is probably the least desirable and most unexpected outcome of an act of sexual intercourse. Yet the act itself continues to remain important as an expression of tenderness, trust, and love. Indeed, the multiple pressures of daily living experienced by middle-aged adults, as well as the irrefutable evidence of physical aging may increase their desire for physical intimacy and for personal reassurance of their continuing sexual attractiveness and competency.

Mace estimates that the entire time occupied in sexual intercourse by the average married couple adds up to the equivalent of about one weekend, or approximately 72 hours, a year.[3] Clearly, this is not enough. Hopefully, throughout their marriage the partners have remained lovers who could excite one another—though this may not be easy while they are working hard at being devoted parents. Because the sexual side of their relationship may now take on added importance, the couple should be encouraged to work at the relationship, to discuss their likes and dislikes regarding techniques, positions, and sex play. Freed from responsibilities to children, they might consider spending a weekend together away from their normal environment, or experimenting with some sensual activities, such as showering together and body massage with warmed oil and fragrant lotions. The nurses can facilitate the couple to consider these activities as a celebration of their love and affection, rather than something frivolous and unimportant.

Incompatibility of sexual drive may appear for the first time during the middle years. It is not uncommon for the woman's libido to increase after menopause, when she no longer fears pregnancy. However, if she devalues herself because of losses related to role change, she may require a lot of her mate's energy to support her, leaving both with depleted reserves to invest in their sexual experience, and predisposing either or both to develop sexual dysfunction. In contrast to women, middle-aged men tend to experience a gradual decline in their sexual interest and activity. Unresolved differences in sexual drive may generate much stress between the partners, and cultural inhibitions unfortunately often result in avoidance of a discussion of these difficulties either between the partners or with health care professionals. Obtaining a good health history continues to be an excellent tool for the nurse both to teach about normal behavior and to gather diagnostic information. Couples who do not intuitively understand that the need for sexual intimacy can be met in a variety of ways may not feel comfortable with anything short of vaginal intercourse unless they are specifically told that other options such as mutual masturbation are normal and healthy, and not indicative of a "poor" sexual relationship. Nurses can provide this kind of sex education.

The developmental stage of their family life causes middle-aged adults to be vulnerable to prolonged periods of separation from their partners. Business trips, visits to adult children, and care-taking responsibilities for ailing parents living in other areas are common realities for many middle-aged couples. The increase in sexual tension during their separation may be problematic for both partners unless they have previously learned how to cope with it. Nurses·are in a unique position to detect this stress and to assist in exploration of alternative coping behavior.

Women apparently tolerate periods of little or no sexual activity better than men.[4] There is still a general belief that men engage in extramarital affairs more frequently than women. However, one recent study found that 36 percent of married women interviewed, as compared with 25 percent in the Kinsey study, had experienced at least one extramarital affair.[5] It is likely that there will be considerable leveling of these differences between the sexes in the next decade or two.

THE SINGLE MIDDLE-AGED ADULT

Relatively little is actually *known* about the sexual behavior of single middle-aged adults. There are plenty of myths. Divorcees are frequently feared and avoided by married women because they are perceived as seductive, promiscuous, and a threat to the marriage. Adults who lose a spouse due to death are frequently "neutered" by family and friends who are unable or unwilling to acknowledge their continuing needs for physical and emotional intimacy. Women who choose to remain single are labeled as "marital rejects" with little or no sexual drive. Men who choose to remain single are perceived as "swingers" with high sex drives requiring a variety of partners. Two middle-aged men who live together are presumed to be gay, although it is a matter of little interest or speculation for two women to live together.

Only one statement about the sexual needs of the single middle-aged adult can be made with any degree of certainty: they clearly exist. Whether the individual deals with them by sublimation, fantasy, cold showers, masturbation, or homosexual or heterosexual activity is a matter of chance, choice, availability, and timing.

The research indicates that nearly all divorced females resume sexual activity following the divorce, as compared with about 50 percent of widows. Widows are usually more financially secure, have feelings of loyalty to the deceased husband, and are subtly inhibited through continuing bonds with in-laws from engaging in sex with other men.[6]

It is essential that nurses acknowledge sexuality as a continuing human drive in all adults. The nurse's listening skills are vital in picking up subtle clues indicating clients' needs to discuss their sexuality, and the nurse's own behavior will establish a climate which either encourages or extinguishes a client's tentative efforts at exploring this sensitive area.

VIGNETTE

Duane is a 45-year-old father of two boys, ages 7 and 9. It is 3 years since his wife died following a very brief illness, and since then he has managed parenting, homemaking, and career responsibilities with remarkable competence. Duane seeks assistance at the local Mental Health Center because he is concerned about his methods of disciplining his sons. The nurse who does the initial interview queries Duane about his own support system. She asks him very matter-of-factly, "How are you meeting your sexual needs?" Duane looks astonished, momentarily confused, and then relieved. He eventually "unloads" a lot of feelings, including guilt, about his continuing need for physical and emotional intimacy.

It seems highly unreasonable to assume that the termination by death, divorce, or separation of a satisfying sexual relationship will not act as a stressor on the person involved. Nurses are becoming increasingly skilled at dealing with other aspects of crises, such as enabling clients to do their grief work, but the sexual needs of the "survivor" frequently are assigned a very low priority or are conspicuous by their absence from nursing-care plans. Nurses, as well as other members of a community, are frequently punitive toward single parents who acknowledge and deal with their sexual drive. Somehow the behavior, no matter how discreet, is interpreted as an affront to the memory of the previous spouse, the moral environment of the children, and the respectability of the neighborhood. The client has a right to be treated with respect, and the nurse has absolutely no responsibility to either condone or reject whatever decisions have been made. The nurse can be helpful in facilitating the client to look at all available options and their outcomes and to consider resources available, and can support the client in taking responsibility for making an informed choice.

This type of problem-solving may bear little relationship to the nurse's formal education. For example, if the problem is inadequate space and/or privacy, the nurse may help the client explore the possibility of making an arrangement with another single parent to swap periodic overnight or weekend child-care responsibilities. For the nurse who gets "rattled" by this type of discussion, it may be helpful to consider it a kind of contingency planning designed to promote and safeguard the health and welfare of both the parent and the child. It is also important for the heterosexual nurse to be clearly aware of her own orientation. It is not safe to conclude that previously married individuals remain heterosexual in their preference, and the nurse will avoid embarrassment for both herself and the client by leaving the options open.

Aside from the adult's own reputation, the major concern about extramarital relationships is usually their effect on the children. The

issue becomes infinitely complicated when the parent has a homosexual preference. The developmental stage of the child will determine what he or she understands about the nature of a parent's
relationship with another adult, and the impact of that relationship
on the parent-child dyad. It is not the purpose of this book to consider childhood experiences in depth, but only to acknowledge that
most parents take very seriously the potential effect of their personal
behavior on their children. Having adult children may increase rather
than decrease the anxiety about engaging in an extramarital relationship, since adult children can be critical and punitive—ostensibly because of loyalty to the other parent, but frequently because of their
own hang-ups. The prerequisite for any attempt by an adult to explain the nature of an intimate relationship to a child is honesty—
honesty with self, with the partner, and with the child, dependent
upon the extent of his ability to understand. Beyond that, nurses
can offer no recipe, since each family situation is unique.

In situations where sexual partners are not available or available
partners are unacceptable, many single middle-aged adults use
masturbation to relieve sexual tension. The women's movement and
the appearance in "respectable" book stores of a variety of publications on "self" and "other" pleasuring have "legitimized" masturbation as an acceptable sexual outlet for both men and women. It
can be a highly gratifying experience, in spite of its common association with a sense of guilt. Nurses can be helpful by acknowledging
that masturbation is a perfectly normal, universal phenomenon, and
"give permission" to clients to practice it (unless their religion forbids it). Nurses need to be sensitive to their own biases, particularly
as they relate to "gimmicks" and "devices," such as body oil and
vibrators. Advice should be limited to matters of safety only, such as
the danger of using an electric vibrator in the bathtub or shower
stall.

Another obvious avenue for single adults to meet their sexual
needs is to engage in a homosexual relationship. Statistics about
the number of American adults having a homosexual preference
remain very unreliable. One should note that there is a degree of
commitment and permanence in many homosexual relationships
equal to or greater than that found in many heterosexual marriages,
particularly if one considers the rising incidence of serial monogamy.
Indeed, the existence of long-term homosexual relationships is a
phenomenological wonder, considering how many social forces are
arrayed against them, as compared with the social supports that
tend to shore up faltering heterosexual marriages. Therefore, to
consider homosexual behavior as a practice engaged in only by single
adults is to discount the reality of many homosexual couples' life

experiences. Again, the women's movement may effect a significant influence on the future prevalence of lesbianism in middle-aged women. Today's young adult women are more likely than their mothers to accept and value a warm, loving, and perhaps sexual relationship with another woman. Considering the differences in life expectancies and the resulting male-female ratio in adult groups, a lesbian relationship may be an increasingly viable option for some single middle-aged women who cannot or prefer not to engage in an intimate relationship with a single male or with someone else's husband.

Some of the concerns of aging in the middle years are common to both a heterosexual and a homosexual orientation. Many gay men verbalize an awareness of the significance of youth and body beauty in a gay partner and a fear of the effects of aging on their ability to attract and retain a significant other. Middle-aged gay men may seek out youthful partners to maintain their own illusion of youth; and while some young gay men prefer the maturity and experience of a middle-aged lover, others may find the visible signs of aging abhorrent in their partners because it confronts them with their own inevitable aging. Regardless of their personal opinions, it is important for nurses to be aware that the gay culture imposes the same kinds of stereotypes on its community as does "straight" society.

Generally speaking, no sexual practices are unique to a homosexual experience. Consequently, there is no specific additional information which nurses need to have when dealing with a client who has a homosexual preference. Sexual behavior, regardless of the gender of one's partner, is as rich and varied as the involved individuals wish it to be.

One final option for the single adult deserves attention. While it may no longer be fashionable to be virgin, there remain some people who choose celibacy as a way of life. They have a right to that choice. Yet because it constitutes a deviation from the accepted norm, it may be perceived as somehow threatening. Many people harbor a good deal of resentment against celibates, especially avowed ones like priests and nuns, and deal with that resentment by making crude jokes, uninformed guesses, or outright statements of disbelief. Just as nurses must avoid the temptation to judge other life-style options, they need to guard against a prejudicial approach to celibates.

UNRESOLVED SEXUAL AROUSAL

Many middle-aged men expect to have some symptoms related to prostate disease. However, there may be another explanation for their low back pain, mild early morning discharge, irritative urinary symptoms, and testicular ache. It is well for the nurse to remember that prolonged petting sessions cause an increased blood supply to the prostate and an increased production of prostatic fluid which, if unrelieved by ejaculation, will result in the discomfort of pelvic congestion, sometimes colorfully known as "blue-balls."

As one author so aptly puts it,

> It appears that the seminal vesicle, reacting to the stimulus of the antici-
> pated sexual activity and ready to perform its function according to nature's
> plan, but having no brains and no morals, accepts disappointment with poor
> grace.[7]

Similarly, women who are frequently or always inorgasmic may suffer from pelvic congestion which manifests itself in nonspecific lower abdominal discomfort. Women who have had children are particularly vulnerable, since they may have residual perineal varicosities and chronic congestion of the pelvic veins.[8]

VIGNETTE
Ursula's routine examination by her gynecologist has revealed no unusual findings to explain her lower abdominal discomfort, general fatigue, and increased irritability. Forty-two years old, with five healthy children and a mother who went through menopause around age 50, she is not manifesting any clinical signs of menopause. Although her Pap tests have been consistently negative, there is a family history of uterine cancer. Ursula expresses concern to the nurse that she may have cancer and that the doctor has chosen not to tell her.

A history of current sexual practice should be taken on clients of either sex who present genitourinary symptoms, to rule out pelvic congestion as the source of their difficulties. Where appropriate, anticipatory guidance can be offered by the nurse to the middle-aged adult who, expecting physical deterioration, diagnoses himself incorrectly. In Ursula's case, a discussion of her current sexual practice would reveal that she has been inorgasmic for the past several months. Because she already fears cancer, she attributes the dysfunction and the attending discomfort of the pelvic congestion to the possibility of a malignancy. The nurse can give Ursula some basic information about the physiology of sexual arousal and the tremendous impact of mind over body in someone who is anxious, fearful, or guilty about their sexual experience. An exploration of the circumstances surrounding the initial inorgasmic experience may lead to further discussion with the couple for the purpose of resolving the dysfunction.

SEXUAL DYSFUNCTION

Men are more vulnerable to sexual dysfunction than women because they must always "perform" and can never merely "permit." A man's ability to function sexually depends on his achieving and maintaining an erection. Masters contends that once a man begins to question his sexual competence, he is 50 percent along the way to impotence.[9] Male dysfunction may also take the form of premature ejaculation or ejaculatory incompetence. Women may experience lack of orgasmic response, vaginismus, or dyspareunia. These categories of dysfunction are well described elsewhere and will not be considered here in detail. They may occur as a result of overindulgence in food or drink, preoccupation with career progress or money-making, mental or physical fatigue, boredom with the monotony of a relationship, drug dependency, and "fear of failure syndrome," leading to a voluntary withdrawal from sexual activity rather than risk an ego-shattering experience.[10] Any of the dysfunctional problems which appear at the time of menopause no doubt existed previously, but the couple becomes more cognizant of them than ever before. Menopause should not be held responsible, and estrogen replacement therapy for the woman will not be the solution.

When sexual dysfunction occurs, it is the relationship itself which is almost always the problem, and consequently the target of treatment. However, any chronic disease is likely to affect the libido, and the middle-aged adult is at risk to many chronic diseases. Diabetes and alcoholism, for example, lead to peripheral neuropathy and resulting impotence; heavy smoking constricts the blood vessels and decreases libido. A large variety of drugs prescribed for health conditions commonly found in middle-aged populations also affect libido and potency. Antihypertensives and antidepressants are frequently cited for their anticholinergic actions, but antihistamines, antispasmodics, sedatives, and tranquilizers are also held responsible for impotence and decreased libido.[11] Health histories should include accurate information about all drugs currently and/or recently taken to rule out drug-induced effects on sexual function. (See sexual history appendix.)

Since the relationship, not one particular client, is seen as owning the problem of sexual dysfunction, there is growing support for treating it using male-female co-therapy teams. Nurses who are comfortable and knowledgeable may choose to become involved as co-therapists. Their basic education and their trust relationship with clients make it logical that nurses should collaborate with physicians and other counselors in treating sexual dysfunction. In addition, they clearly have a responsibility to be involved in case-finding and referral. Rosenthal cites particular advantages for including a female therapist when treating a dysfunctional couple.[12] The female co-therapist is a new authority figure who serves as an identification model for the woman client. Specific permission is given by both the male and female authority figures to both clients to allow them to enjoy their sexuality and sensuality. This contributes to their ability to incorporate on an emotional level what they may already know on an intellectual level. With the increasing concern for assuring that the public will be safeguarded from charlatans and quacks practicing sex therapy, nurses who wish to develop this area of specialization should pursue additional preparation in accredited programs, as well as negotiate for adequate supervision of their practice from competent peers.

BIBLIOGRAPHY

1   Pfeiffer, Eric, and G. C. Davis: "Determinants of Sexual Behavior in Middle and Old Age," *J. Amer. Geriat. Soc.*, 20:151-158, 1972.

2   Hunt, Morton: *Sexual Behavior in the 1970's*, Playboy Press, Chicago, 1974.

3   Mace, David, and Vera Mace: "The Joy of Human Sexuality in Marriage," *J. Sex Education Ther.*, 2:35-41, 1975.

4   Pomeroy, Wardell B., and Cornelia V. Christenson: *Characteristics of Male and Female Sexual Responses*, Study Guide No. 4, SIECUS, New York, 1967.

5   Athanasiou, Robert: "Questionnaire," *Psychology Today*, July 1970, pp. 37-52.

6   Gebhardt, Paul H.: "Heterosexual Behavior," Lecture delivered at Institute for Sex Research (Summer Program 1974), Bloomington, University of Indiana, June 19, 1974.

7   Lehfeldt, Hans: "Pelvic Pain After Petting," *Med. Aspects Human Sexuality*, 3 (9): 47, 1969.

8   Kogan, Benjamin A.: *Human Sexual Expression*, Harcourt Brace Jovanovich, Inc., New York, 1973.

9   Masters, William: "Human Sexuality," Lecture delivered at workshop at Oasis Midwest Center for Human Potential, Chicago, May 19, 1974.

10 Rubin, Isadore: *Sexual Life in the Later Years*, Study Guide No. 12, SIECUS, New York, 1970.

11 Woods, James S.: "Drug Effects on Human Sexual Behavior," in *Human Sexuality in Health and Illness*, pp. 175-191, The C. V. Mosby Company, St. Louis, 1975.

12 Rosenthal, Saul H., and Chauncey F. Rosenthal: "Joint Sexual Counseling," *Southern Med. J.*, 68 (1): 46-48, 1975.

13 Barbach, Lonnie Garfield: *For Yourself: The Fulfillment of Female Sexuality*, Anchor Books, Doubleday & Company, Inc., Garden City, N.Y., 1976.

14 Colton, Helen: *Sex After the Sexual Revolution*, Association Press, New York, 1972.

15   Comfort, Alex: *The Joy of Sex*, Crown Publishers, Inc., New York, 1972.

16   Falk, Ruth: *Women Loving*, Random House, Inc., New York, 1975.

17   Kaplan, Helen Singer: *The New Sex Therapy*, Brunner/Mazel, Inc., New York, 1974.

18   Kline-Graber, Georgia, and Benjamin Graber: *Woman's Orgasm*, The Bobbs-Merrill Co., Inc., Indianapolis, 1975.

19   Lee, Ronald D., Frank Melleno, and Robert Mullis: *Gay Men Speak*, Multi-Media Resource Center, San Francisco, 1973.

20   Martin, Del, and Phyllis Lyon: *Lesbian Love and Liberation*, Multi-Media Resource Center, San Francisco, 1973.

21   McIlvenna, Ted, and Herb Vandervoort: *You Can Last Longer*, Multi-Media Resource Center, San Francisco, 1972.

22   O'Neill, Nena, and George O'Neill: *Open Marriage*, Avon Books Division, The Hearst Corporation, New York, 1972.

23   Rimmer, Robert H.: *Adventures in Loving*, Signet Books, New American Library, Inc., New York, 1973.

24   Rush, Anne Kent: *Getting Clear: Body Work for Women*, Random House, Inc. Booksworks, New York, 1973.

25   Smith, Carolyn, Toni Ayres, and Maggie Rubenstein: *Getting in Touch: Self Sexuality for Women*, Multi-Media Resource Center, San Francisco, 1972.

26   Wabrek, Carolyn J., and Alan J. Wabreck: "Sexual Difficulties and the Importance of the Relationship," *Nursing Digest*, 111 (6): 44-45, 1975.

27   Weinberg, George: *Society and the Healthy Homosexual*, St. Martin's Press, Inc., New York, 1972.

CHAPTER 10

Male and Female Menopause

The term "change of life" is frequently applied to both menopause and climacterium. *Menopause*, which occurs only in women, means the cessation of the menses. *Climacterium*, which occurs in both sexes, means the loss of ability to reproduce. For a woman, the menopause and climacterium occur together. For a man, the climacterium occurs about 20 years later than for a woman, for he does not lose his ability to reproduce until his seventies or eighties. However, there is a male reaction, psychosocial rather than physiological, which resembles the female menopause and occurs at about the same time; this may be referred to as the "pseudo-climacterium," or the "male menopause."

PHYSIOLOGICAL CHANGES IN FEMALE MENOPAUSE
Menopause has received very little attention and is almost ignored in nursing literature. Some nurses feel that it is not a health problem and therefore they need not be concerned about it. Some feel it should be handled exclusively by the physician. Some feel nothing can be done about it, and therefore it is to be ignored. None of these opinions is correct. Menopause is not a pathological state, but

a normal physiological event in a woman's life and development. It is an event, however, which often brings with it problems that the nurse can help with and for which she can provide anticipatory guidance.

Menopause represents a transitional phase in a woman's life—a phase of adjustment to the waning potential of the ovary—which takes place over a period of about 15 years, between approximately 45 and 60 years of age, and is the counterpart of puberty.[1] A premature menopause, one that takes place before the age of 40, occurs in only about 8 percent of women. During this time, the woman is neither predictably sterile nor frigid. The key physical change is permanent and irreversible atrophy of the ovaries, accompanied by a corresponding decline in estrogen and progesterone production. With the cessation of ovulation, it has been established that estrogenic production in the human female does not completely disappear. Studies[2,3] of vaginal smears have shown an estrogenic effect to persist for a decade or more beyond the menopause in nearly 80 percent of all postmenopausal women. One study found that 40 percent of post menopausal women maintain moderate levels of estrogenic activity during the remaining years of life.[3] This residual estrogen is produced by the adrenal gland, the ovarian stromal cells which have the capacity for steroidogenesis, and perhaps from an unknown source yet to be determined.[1]

Because an individual's potential for functioning in a satisfactory sexual relationship is so closely involved with the perception of one's body as sensuous and attractive, it is important to consider the visible effect on the body of the gradually diminishing ovarian function. Some signs precede menopause. For example, the breasts may become turgid and tender and even increase in size, probably as a result of the unmodified effect of the estrogen during anovulatory cycles, and also, it is thought, because of increased pituitary stimulation. At this time, cystic mastitis or other fibrocystic conditions of the breasts may develop or grow worse.[4]

Widespread changes also occur in the integument with estrogen deprivation and aging. The skin as a whole becomes thinner and loses elasticity and turgor. Scaling and wrinkles gradually appear, sending flocks of women to cosmetic counters to purchase false hope in the form of estrogen creams and lotions. After menopause, as fat, glandular tissue, and tone decrease, buttocks and breasts actually shrink and droop. The nipples become smaller and lose their erectile character.

The hot flush or flash is the sure sign of the menopausal syndrome, as it occurs only in this instance. Hot flashes may occur over a period of from 1 to 10 years, and in some women appear before the menopause is definitely established, during the time when the estrogen levels are known to fluctuate. They gradually begin as a sensation of warmth over the upper part of the chest and characteristically spread, wave-like, over the neck, face, and upper extremities. They appear with unpredictable suddenness and are often followed by profuse perspiration and chilliness.[1] They are especially disturbing at night, interfering with sleep; perspiration may be so drenching as to require a change of bedclothes. The frequency and severity are subject to wide variation. Flushes and sweats are usually more severe in anxious women and are intensified by excitement or stress. Other vasomotor symptoms include numbness and tingling, cold hands and feet, vertigo, and palpitations. The precise mechanism for the vasomotor symptoms is uncertain. Evidence points to a disturbance in the equilibrium between the hypothalamus and the autonomic nervous system, both of which apparently become conditioned to a high estrogen level and then react to its decline.

Atrophic vaginitis occurs more commonly some years after menopause begins. Because of estrogen insufficiency, the vaginal epithelium eventually becomes pale and dry due to decreasing vascularity and atrophy of the mucous membrane. The loose purple rugae of the vaginal walls becomes thin, pale, and fragile and "sweats" less lubricant during sexual arousal, especially if the woman neither masturbates nor has intercourse more than once or twice a month. There may be pain on penetration. The vaginal mucosa is easily eroded and may bleed or develop adhesions. The normally acidic vaginal secretions become alkaline or only slightly acidic, thus increasing susceptibility to infection, even by organisms of normally low virulence. The predominating symptoms of senile vaginitis reported by women clients are discharge, itching, burning, and dyspareunia, or painful intercourse.

Many women do not realize that these changes are normal and the problems that can result can be remedied with medication. Thus if the nurse prepares the premenopausal woman for these changes, especially the possibility that she may experience painful intercourse, the client will not blame herself for not being able to respond to her partner, or feel she is frigid or not able to be sexually active anymore. She will be alert to the probable cause and will seek out medical advice at that time.

Atrophic changes due to estrogen deficiency also cause the supporting structures of the uterus, bladder, and rectum to lose tone and strength, favoring the development of uterine prolapse, cystocele, and rectocele, especially in women who have borne children. Urinary symptoms such as frequency, urgency, and burning on urination and defective bladder control may send women to consult their doctors.

Since a woman client is particularly susceptible to bladder infections at this time, it is important for the nurse to review good personal hygiene, so that she can avoid bladder infections whenever possible.

During menopause, menstrual periods commonly become shorter, with decreased flow, and may vary in frequency, at times skipping 1 or more months. However, all kinds of menstrual disturbance may herald the menopause: menorrhagia, metrorrhagia, hypomenorrhea, polymenorrhea, and oligomenorrhea. Of major concern to sexually active women is the question of how long following the cessation of menstruation is it safe to discard birth control. Pregnancy has occurred up to age 50.[5] Occasionally an ovulatory cycle will occur while the woman is still menstruating. Taking oral contraceptives will not postpone the beginning of menopause, which is genetically determined, but will simply mask it. If a woman is taking the pill, she will not menstruate if she is menopausal when the drug is stopped. One gynecologist recommends that women discontinue the pill at age 44. If normal menses resume spontaneously within 3 months, the woman would resume taking the pill for another 9 months. She then goes off the pill for 3 months and repeats the cycle. If no menstrual period occurs during this time, she is assumed to be menopausal.[6] Six months following the cessation of menstruation is a reasonably safe time to discontinue birth control. Most gynecologists recommend the use of some form of birth control other than oral contraceptives during these months as an extra precautionary measure. It is important that unwanted pregnancies be avoided for the sake of both mother and child. The 40-year-old mother is considered high risk because of her age; and the incidence of abnormal births in this group, particularly of children with Down's syndrome, is very high.

The physiological signs of aging may be very difficult for a woman to accept, especially in view of today's emphasis on youth and the competition which she may feel from younger members of her sex. For a woman who cannot accept a fading of physical allure and youthfulness, and whose sense of self-worth derives from a need to have her body admired, a sense of loss will inevitably follow as the aging process begins to become more visible and public. Similarly, the loss of generative power which accompanies menopause may precipitate a full-blown grief reaction in the woman whose sense of femininity is intimately tied to her fertility, regardless of her marital status.

ESTROGEN-REPLACEMENT THERAPY
The use of estrogens during and after menopause is controversial. Some physicians feel that menopause, with its accompanying reduc-

tion in estrogen, is a natural process not to be tampered with; others hold that it is a deficiency state, to be treated in order to prevent the acceleration of aging.[7] In our youth-and-beauty-centered culture, some women are tricked into believing that estrogen-replacement therapy will keep them forever young. This, of course, is a myth. Aging cannot be prevented by estrogens alone; too many other factors are involved.

Coronary heart disease below the age of 40 appears in fifteen men to one woman. In the total population, however, the difference drops sharply; the disease occurs in only two or three men to one woman.[6] Its incidence in women, therefore, rises markedly after menopause. Is it the loss of estrogen in postmenopausal women which accounts for this?

According to one view, estrogen replacement protects women from coronary artery disease, and there is some support for this in the fact that women seem to be protected from the disease while their estrogen is high and are more susceptible to it later, after menopause, when their estrogen has markedly decreased. According to Doctors Graber and Barber, however, there are no valid studies which demonstrate that estrogens prevent the coronary heart disease.[8] Another disease, senile osteoporosis, usually occurs in women 10 or more years after menopause. This is manifested by a decrease in stature and the development of dorsal kyphosis, or "dowager hump," and is accompanied by bone pain and fractures due to decalcification and decrease in bone mass. Estrogen, and particularly estrogen replacement, does appear to have some influence on bone density for a period of time. However, low-protein and low-calcium diets and the sedentary life often led by aging women appear to be more significant factors in this disease than the presence or absence of estrogen.[8]

In any event, there are many cases in which estrogen therapy is contraindicated: first, women who have a history of cancer, particularly uterine, genital, or breast, since malignant growths can easily be triggered in genetically susceptible women;[8] secondly, women with a history of hypertension, edema due to congestive heart failure, diabetes, uterine fibroids, thromboembolism, abnormal liver function, and any acute inflammatory disease such as rheumatism.[4]

Three major symptoms of menopause—flushes and sweats, atrophic vaginitis, and insomnia—can be relieved by estrogen. Estrogen is an excellent drug, and under certain conditions it can be very successfully used. However, clients need to be aware of the pluses and minuses of this type of therapy. The aim of estrogen therapy should be to control the symptoms as rapidly as possible with as little medication as possible.

PSYCHOSOCIAL ASPECTS OF FEMALE MENOPAUSE

If we think of this period as it has been defined, as a transition from one period of life to another and the counterpart of puberty, it is easy to see that many women may find difficulties in making the adjustment. The physiological signs of aging may be very difficult for many a woman to accept, particularly a woman who, influenced by the exaggerated American emphasis on youth, has become addicted to having her body admired. And for any woman, the recognition that she has lost her generative power is bound to be a milestone. This is especially true if she feels that that power is the essence of her femininity, and if she has devoted the major share of her energy to efforts to stay young and physically attractive, instead of looking forward to the challenges, services, and rewards which inevitably accompany maturity, if she will only look for them. The nurse can do much to help her clients make this transition with grace.

Some women, overwhelmed by menopause as a sign of their own mortality, may feel cheated and angry as they realize that they have given a large portion of their lives to childbearing and childrearing, and that their children are now on the point of leaving home to live their own lives. For such a woman, the adjustment of being "alone together" with her husband may require as much effort as did the initial adjustment to marriage.[9] Not only can the nurse help to show her that she has much to look forward to in the new situation; the nurse can also help the husband to understand and be sympathetic with his wife's point of view.

The husband can be told that during menopause, his wife may need more recreation, amusement, and rest than usual. She may need to be told more that she's loved and appreciated and that she is sexually satisfying. It may be helpful for the husband to show more interest in birthdays and anniversaries. Sometimes, when she is feeling blue, it may be helpful to go to a movie or to pitch in to do the household chores together. A long-wished-for trip might also help the wife better cope with menopause.[10]

It is interesting to note that, in a study by Neugarten[11] of 100 women between the ages of 45 and 55, in which they were asked to list the fears they had of middle age, menopause did not rank very high. Of greatest concern was widowhood. Generally, women feared 'getting older," "lack of energy," and "poor health or illness." As to menopause, the best thing was either not worrying about pregnancy or not having to bother any more with menstruation; the worst was not knowing what to expect, the pain and discomfort of menopause, and its indication that they were growing older. A most significant finding of this study was that the women concerned were extremely eager to discuss menopause and very curious about it. We give little social support to menopausal women as compared with the very great amount we give to pregnant women.

Many women are reluctant to bring up menopause with a male doctor because they are afraid he will brush the topic off as unimportant. They will talk much more freely with another woman. She should listen. She should be an attentive, careful, encouraging listener. A listening attitude is very important because many times the client is validating that what she is experiencing is normal.[12] The nurse can give this assurance. Also, she can encourage the woman to relax and to go along with, rather than fight, changes in body rhythms. Many women in the menopause feel bursting with energy one day, and as if they were getting over a bad flu attack the next; the nurse can suggest some rearrangement of their schedules so that they can tackle heavy jobs on the former days and rest up on the latter. Since insomnia is common in this period, she can advise them to get up in the night and do something such as write letters or read until they begin to feel sleepy again, instead of wearing themselves out tossing and turning. For many clients, this is an excellent time to pick up some outside activities; the nurse can suggest beginning shopping or luncheon engagements with friends, volunteer work, concerts, or short trips, though these should be so planned that clients do not wear themselves out. She might also point out the advantages of taking naps when they feel like it and have the chance.

One myth of menopause the nurse can dispel is that it ends a woman's interest and participation in a regular sexual relationship. In fact, the function of the ovary has little to do with either libido or orgasm. It is true that a woman's view of herself as a lovable, sexually desirable partner may be dependent on her own body image, or her own sense of self-esteem, or both, and if either of these is diminished, her libido is bound to be affected also. Pfeiffer also suggests that the extent of an aging woman's sexual activity and interest depends heavily on the availability to her of a socially sanctioned, sexually capable partner.[13] Physiologically, however, there is no reason why a woman may not engage in sexual activity well into her advanced years. Opportunity for regular sexual expression (at least once a week) is important to maintain lubrication and distensibility, and the vagina is not discriminatory as to the source of that stimulation, whether it be self- or other-initiated. If there is genital discomfort and/or senile vaginitis, local application of estrogen cream or suppositories will restore the vaginal epithelium to its former thickness and reduce the symptoms. Positive feelings about oneself, the opportunity to be sexually active, and habit are the key to sexual satisfaction.

PHYSIOLOGICAL CHANGES OF MALE MENOPAUSE

There needs to be a differentiation made between what happens to a man in his fifties and what happens to a man in his seventies. Testosterone levels reach their peak at about age 20 in the male. After that age, they begin dropping, though there is a plateau between the ages of 40 and 60. After 60, they continue to drop until at about age 70 they become so low that they effect a serious decline in libido and sexual capacity, as well as muscular strength and aggressiveness. At this time, climacterium, the man may experience hot flashes, sweating attacks, anxiety, depression, and nightmares. He may also become forgetful and even forget where he is or what he is doing. Since this occurs 20 years later than in the female, and the individual is in his seventies, the forgetfulness is often times just attributed to hardening of the arteries. While this is true, it may not account for all the forgetfulness.

There is disagreement among the "experts" as to whether or not there is a discrete phenomenon known as the male menopause. The middle-aged man may experience a gradually diminishing virility and a slackening of his ability to perform sexually, a syndrome particularly distressing to men who have depended on sexual prowess to sustain their sense of masculinity and youthfulness. Change in the sexual response cycle reflects the general slowing-down effect of normal aging on other parts of the musculoskeletal system. The sex flush decreases, erection takes longer to achieve, ejaculation is less forceful and shorter in duration, and the refractory period may increase. However, with regular sexual expression and a stimulating sexual climate, the healthy man's sexual capacity should extend well into the 80-year level. Again, it is critical to remember that there is much individual variation. A 47-year-old may enjoy a half-hour refractory period while a 32-year-old may require 8 to 12 hours. There is no national norm against which all men can measure their sexual behavior.

However, those symptoms which are associated with male menopause, such as moodiness, impatience, worry, touchiness, headaches, and hypochondria,[14] are often attributed to the fact that the middle-aged man is worried about competition from younger men, decreasing opportunities for job changes and/or advancement, and pressure to provide for retirement while maintaining the present standard of living.

Whether or not a man is diagnosed and treated for male menopause depends on the frame of reference of the physician from whom he seeks care. Borderline testosterone titers are associated with decreasing libido, but the titer is also known to fluctuate according to increased stress and loss of self-esteem.

VIGNETTE

Nathaniel, age 52, has been feeling generally run-down. He is aware that his sexual drive has decreased markedly over the past year. Once or twice he has been impotent. He is feeling depressed because he has reached his maximum earning potential as a semi-skilled laborer, and he worries about financing his daughter's upcoming wedding. There is a history of adult-onset diabetes in Nathaniel's family.

Given that the findings on his medical exam and lab tests are within normal limits, except for a borderline testosterone level, Nathaniel may be seen as pre-morbid in whatever area of specialization his physician practices. For example, a psychiatrist may interpret reduced libido as a part of depression due to his life experiences and prescribe psychotherapy. An internist may see it as a precursor of diabetes and prescribe diet modification and weight loss. An endocrinologist may prescribe testosterone to elevate the libido. In all probability, any intervention that improves Nathaniel's general state of health and induces a sense of well-being will be effective in causing an increased libido, because men are so vulnerable to suggestion of sexual failure and are easily locked into a spiral of self-defeat. The important thing for nurses to be aware of is the complexity of the syndrome and the variety of approaches to treatment. Testosterone can be prescribed for symptomatic purposes; however it is not usually prescribed for prolonged periods since it tends to accelerate atherosclerosis or heart disease.[15] Nurses need to bear in mind that there are expectations related to socioeconomic status and culture which may exacerbate Nathaniel's problem. It is not uncommon for blue-collar workers of all ages to expect to be sexually very active and to perceive any reduction or interruption in that activity as a serious threat to their health.[16] Nurses need to be alert and responsive to this type of concern.

PSYCHOSOCIAL ASPECTS OF MALE MENOPAUSE

After the age of 50, depression and self-destructive behavior significantly increase in males; 25 percent of all divorces and remarriages involve middle-aged males.[15] At this time many men desire and feel the need of greater stimulation in all areas of their lives, including sex, and seek out younger partners to experience it. The man often is not aware that his desire may be the result of normal reduction at his age in his ability to see, hear, smell, and experience sexual and sensual stimulation. It is equally important for the man to understand himself and for his wife to understand him. This is often asking a good deal. The wife also may be experiencing menopause, and be in need of understanding and support herself. It is not only possible, but easy, for great misunderstandings to arise between them; the nurse may do much to dispel these misunderstandings if she is sympathetic with both those caught in the situation.

We have already pointed out that the nurse can help to show the woman that middle age is not an end, but a new beginning. She can do the same thing for the man. Something has been lost, yes; but lost normally and inevitably in the process of moving toward potential gain. At this time, a man may naturally take stock of what he has accomplished with his life, and he may not feel satisfied; he may perceive new horizons; he may want to do his "own thing." An understanding wife can sympathize and encourage. A man may turn to alcohol or to hypochondria. Again, an understanding wife (and the nurse can help her to be understanding) can try to distract her husband from these undesirable outlets by providing variety and excitement. Our society teaches women, for example, how to whet their husbands' appetites at the dinner table, but not in bed; the nurse may help an uninstructed wife here. She can certainly point out the importance of giving the husband compliments rather than criticism and a sympathetic ear rather than an angry voice at this period of his life. To take a very trivial instance, if the husband falls asleep in front of the television after dinner, the wife should not make a scene about it but understand that he may simply need a nap. At this time of life, some men panic. But there is no more need for a man to panic because he has reached an inevitable and normal stage of his life which means a change, than there is for a theater audience to get up and go home when the curtain falls after the first act. There is much for him to look forward to as it rises on a new stage set.

ANTICIPATORY GUIDANCE AND MENOPAUSE

Since we are all human, men and women alike, we all deal in different ways, and with varying degrees of success, with the change of life. The nurse, by providing anticipatory guidance, can help her clients successfully cope with menopause. She can listen, and she can provide suggestions and reassurance. Some people choose to deal with the change of life by denying it and turning their attention to other things. This method might be quite successful, as in the case of a teacher who decides it is the right time for him to write a book on a subject he has always wanted to treat. It might be unsuccessful, as in the case of a man who overcompensates by sexual conquests and thereby breaks up a long-standing, happy marriage at the cost of great pain to wife and children; or of a woman who feels a compulsion to spend large amounts of money on surgery to restore the youthful appearance it is impossible for her to maintain. In these cases intervention and referral may be appropriate by the nurse.[17]

But many middle adults can be helped to see the change of life for what it is: inevitable, hopeful, and the opportunity to make progress in freeing oneself from childish self-centeredness; the opportunity to grow not only old, but mature, wise, and happy; and the opportunity to become interested in, and to serve, others.

BIBLIOGRAPHY

1 Cali, Robert W.: "Management of the Climacteric and Postmenopausal Woman," *Med. Clinics N. Amer.*, **56** (3):789-800, 1972.

2 Masukawa, T.: "Vaginal Smears in Women Past 40 Years of Age with Emphasis on Their Remaining Hormonal Activity," *Obstet. Gynecol.*, 16:407-413, 1960.

3 McLennan, M. T., and C. E. McLennan: "Estrogenic Status of Menstruating and Menopausal Women Assessed by Cervico-Vaginal Smears," *Obstet. Gynecol.*, 37:325-331, 1971.

4 *A Clinical Guide to Menopause and the Post-Menopause*, Ayerst Laboratories, New York, 1968.

5. Claman, A. D., David Swartz, R. A. H. Kinch, and N. B. Hirt: "Panel Discussion: Sexual Difficulties After 50: General Discussion," *Can. Med. Assoc. J.*, 94:215-217, 1966.

6 Bender, S.: "Is Your Menopause Really Necessary?" *Nursing Mirror*, 133(1): 30-31, 1971.

7 Kaste, Nathan: "Estrogens and the Menopause," *J. Amer. Med. Assoc.*, 227:318-319, 1974.

8 Graber, Edward A., and Hugh R. K. Barber: "The Case For and Against Estrogen Therapy," *Amer. J. Nursing*, 75:1766-1771, 1975.

9 Galloway, Karen: "The Change of Life," *Amer. J. Nursing*, 75:1006-1011, 1975.

10 The Retirement Council (Editor and Pub.): *Better Health After Fifty*, American Heritage Publishing Co., Inc., New York, 1964.

11 Neugarten, Bernice L.: "The Awareness of Middle Age," in Roger Owen (ed.), *Middle Age*, British Broadcasting Corporation, London, 1967.

12 McEwan, J. A.: "Menopause: Myths and Medicine," *Nursing Times*, **69:** 1483-1484, 1973.

13 Pfeiffer, Eric, Adriaan Verwoerdt, and Glenn C. Davis: "Sexual Behavior in the Middle Life," *Amer. J. Psychiat.*, 128(10)1262-1267, 1972.

14 Rubin, T.: "Male Menopause," *Ladies Home Journal*, Nov. 1971, p. 52.

15 Allen, G.: "Do Men Go Through a Change of Life?" *Family Health*, Nov. 1972, pp. 20-23.

16 LeMasters, E. E.: *Blue Collar Aristocrats*, University of Wisconsin Press, Madison, 1975.

17 Marmor, J.: "The Crisis of Middle Age," *R.N.*, 30(11):63-68, 1967.

18 Dresen, Sheila: "The Full Life," *Amer. J. Nursing*, 75:1008-1011, 1976.

19 Hirt, Norman: "Sexual Difficulties After 50: The Psychiatrist's View," *Can. Med. Assoc. J.*, **94**:213-214, 1966.
20 Kase, Nathan: "Estrogens and the Menopause," *J. Amer. Med. Assoc.*, **227**:318-319, 1974.
21 Kinch, R. A. H.: "Sexual Difficulties After 50: The Gynecologist's View," *Can. Med. Assoc. J.*, **94**:211-212, 1966.
22 Lear, M. W.: "Is There a Male Menopause?" *New York Times Magazine*, Jan 28, 1973, pp. 10-11.
23 Ryan, K. J., and D. C. Gibson (eds.): *Menopause and Aging*, Summary Report and Selected Papers from a Research Conference, May 1971, Hot Springs, Ark., DHEW Publication (NIH) No. 73-319, Bethesda, Md., Public Health Service, 1973.
24 Steiner, Betty W.: "The Crisis of Middle Age," *CMA J.*, **109**:1017-1027, 1973.
25 Swartz, David: "Sexual Difficulties After 50: The Urologist's View," *Can. Med. Assoc. J.*, **94**:208-210, 1966.

Living Sensibly

The Older Adult

PART THREE

CHAPTER 11

Older Adulthood–
An Overview

Aging adults continue to grow until the moment of death. Aging is not an illness, but a gradual slowing down. It involves physiological, mental, emotional, and physical changes which will differ markedly in individuals in extent and pace. Aging cannot be stopped, but it can be retarded by good preventive health care and by the proper nutrition, exercise, and rest.

Many myths about aging exist. Five myths, popularly and erroneously held, will be discussed before proceeding factually and realistically with the topic of aging.[1]

The first myth of aging is that of tranquility. It presents old age as a time of idyllic serenity when the old enjoy the fruits of their labors. At first glance it might seem a pity that this is only a myth, but a wiser second thought would show that the continuing emotional, physical, and financial problems, which exist for the elderly as they do for all of us at all periods, are simply a part of life and are necessary to keep old people from stagnation and senility.

The second myth, an unpleasant contrasting one, is that of senility. This label is not an actual medical term, but one often and carelessly used to indicate forgetfulness and mental confusion, or "second childhood." It is certainly true that for some persons brain deterioration due to cerebral arteriosclerosis appears at this age; it is not true that all old persons are senile.

The third is the myth of unproductivity. It is assumed erroneously that older adults can no longer be productive on a job, or be active socially, or be creative. For some older persons, again, this may be true if they have a chronic debilitating disease. However, many older adults remain productive as evidenced by the fact that the 1971 Bureau of Labor statistics showed 780,000 persons over 65 years of age employed full time in America, and 1,257,000 part-time.

The fourth myth is that the elderly resist change. It is true that character is remarkably stable in this age group. But their acceptance of or resistance to change depends far more on life-long personality traits than on anything inherent in this period. When examined, an act which might be considered reactionary may be the result of economic pressure; for instance, if elderly people voted against a new highway assessment or a new school building, the reason might well be their knowledge that their fixed income would not allow them to pay the higher taxes which the proposal would call for.

Finally, the myth exists that aging is a matter of pure chronology, or that one 80-year-old has aged approximately as much in all ways as another. Nothing could be further from the truth. There are large disparities between physiological, psychological, chronological, and social ages; people age at widely different rates, and people become more divergent with age. Thus, one 80-year-old may conform to the *stereotype* for that age; another in health, appearance, activity, and mental acuity might pass for a person of 60.

PHYSIOLOGICAL CHANGES IN THE OLDER ADULT

In the older adult years, anatomical-physiological-biochemical changes occur in the normal process of aging; at the same time, other changes may occur in the process of disease. Disease is considered abnormal; aging is considered normal. Difficulty may arise in deciding to which cause a given symptom should be ascribed. For example, blood pressure, especially systolic pressure, increases with age; increase in blood pressure is also a symptom of heart disease. In current medical practice, conditions which are readily detected and easily treated often are identified as diseases; conditions which are perhaps difficult to identify or which might call for hazardous therapy may be ascribed to old age and are left alone. Nurses need to be observant of, sensitive to, and creative with older clients. Their knowledge of diseases must be supplemented with knowledge of aging, which is a process of infinite variety.

With aging, bone density and strength decrease. The ligaments become calcified and muscular weakness may be noted, resulting in fractures and osteoporosis. Difficulty with elimination may occur. Postural changes are not uncommon, particularly stooped back (kyphosis). Arthritis and stiffening of the joints may impair mobility.

There is a decrease in the production of digestive juices and of muscle tone in the stomach and intestines, a decline in the senses of taste and smell, and often loss of teeth. Basal metabolism decreases. Constipation, poor appetite, and malnutrition can result, and changes in food habits can cause either gain or loss in weight.

The muscle tone of the bladder and of the muscle controlling urination decreases; there is a decline in the hormonal secretions in both males and females and enlargement of the prostate gland in males. These changes can result in urinary retention, incontinence, and urinary dribbling. There may also be a decrease in the size of the vaginal opening with dryness of the vagina, due to the decline in estrogen.

Decrease in the elasticity of blood vessels and decreased cardiac output are another concomitant of old age. Deposits of fat-like substances in the walls of the vessels may contribute to arteriosclerosis, hypertension, and other types of heart trouble. Dizziness may occur as a result of getting up too quickly from a sitting or lying position, and a decrease in the circulation of the blood to the brain may also result in forgetfulness.

There is also a decrease in the speed of conduction of nerve impulses, which usually results in a slower reaction time. The rigidity of the bones of the middle ear increases, and there may be a gradual hearing loss, especially of higher tones. As a result, older adults may find it difficult to locate or identify sounds or to understand group conversations; for this reason, they sometimes fail to enjoy, and then stay away from, social occasions, and may develop some tinge of suspicion, since they may hear only part of what is being said. Many elderly complain that they can "hear" but cannot "understand" speech.[2]

Changes occur also in the eye. Loss of elasticity in the lens, reduction in pupil size, and decline in the speed of adjustment to light mean that the older adults may need more light to conduct the tasks of daily living.[3] It may be hard to distinguish colors. Glasses are often needed for reading. Night driving may become difficult, or even dangerous.

Lastly, there is a loss of fatty tissue and skin elasticity, a decrease in the lubrication secretions of the skin, and an increase in the fragility of the blood vessels. The result may be chilliness due to the decreased ability of the body to regulate temperature, dry and itchy skin, and easy bruising.

Along with these physiological changes, there may be other

obvious changes in appearance. The nose appears elongated, a double or triple chin develops, the skin wrinkles, the shoulders stoop, and the abdomen bulges and droops. The nails of the hands and feet become thick, tough, and brittle. A woman's breasts become flabby and droop. While not all older adults show these signs of aging, nor do all of them occur simultaneously, they are so common that sooner or later all elderly persons recognize some of them in themselves. Here, the nurse can provide anticipatory guidance and help clients view these changes as normal. Many people, victims perhaps of our American overemphasis on youth and glamor, "fight" aging and waste money, time, and hope trying to resist the inevitable; the nurse may help them to accept it.

These changes of aging, collected all together, make a formidable list. But it is to be remembered that aging in a highly individual matter. Some changes may indeed cause discomfort to some clients, but many will pass practically unnoticed or require only slight adjustment. The nurse can give clients peace of mind by informing them that this or that symptom means normal aging, and not necessarily disease, and that aging is the normal human condition to which no one is immune. If these changes are taken with good sense and good humor, there is no reason for the older adult to be distressed or disturbed by them.

INTELLECTUAL CHANGES

As is true in other areas of aging, there are marked individual variations in mental decline. There is no one age when it begins and no specific pattern characteristic of all older adults. It is sometimes assumed that physical decline is accompanied by mental decline; in some instances this is true, in others it is not. In general, persons of high intellectual capacity experience less decrease in mental efficiency than those of low intellectual capacity. Environmental stimulation can greatly retard the rate of decline, an encouraging factor since to some extent this is under the control of the person involved. Those who continue to "work" show better brain functioning and perform better on intelligence tests than those who are idle. "Work" is here to be taken in the broadest sense, encompassing all kinds of mental activity, not merely in the narrow sense of continuing to hold a given job.

It is now believed that older adulthood is accompanied by less mental decline than was formerly thought.[4] However, the whole area of mental change is controversial with very little real evidence to go on, and much of the sampling which has been done in this field is now suspect. Most older adults are not practiced in standardized testing, with which today's young children very early become familiar. Moreover, older adults are often rather distrustful of new testing methods and often refuse to submit to them. Thus many samples are not representative and do not present an accurate picture. In order truly to measure the decline of mental abilities with age, we need longitudinal studies: accurate measurements of persons at their peak, and continuous subsequent measurements as they age. Few such studies exist. It is to be noted, then, that questions exist as to the adequacy of the evidence on which the following generalizations are based.

Old persons are more cautious about learning and need more time to integrate their responses than young ones. They are less capable of dealing with new material. In both deductive and inductive reasoning, it takes them longer to reach a conclusion (partly, perhaps, as a result of the tendency toward increased caution with increasing age). Significant creative achievements are less common among older adults than among younger ones, and many lack the capacity for or interest in creative thinking.[5] (However, the poet Robert Frost, the playwright George Bernard Shaw, the philosopher Bertrand Russell, and the artists Georgia O'Keefe and Grandma Moses were still going strong in their late eighties or even nineties. While it is unlikely that the nurse's clients will include geniuses like this, you never know!)

Older adults tend to have a poor memory for recent events, but a good memory for remote ones.[5] This may be partly due to the fact that they have little motivation to remember recent events, and partly due to lack of attentiveness. Age affects recall more than it does recognition. Many older people use cues—especially visual, auditory, and kinesthetic ones—to aid their ability to recall. Mental rigidity sometimes appears in middle age and intensifies with increasing years. The cause may be that it is more difficult for the elderly to learn new concepts, or that loyalty to old values and methods forbids abandoning them for new ones, or both.

On the other hand, Neugarten has shown that, though cognitive processes decline with age, competence in role performance and interpersonal skills shows little or no decrease.[6] It is important for the nurse to emphasize to elderly clients that their life experience is, accordingly, a real asset of their age.

EMOTIONAL CHANGES

The self-concept ("Who am I?") alters little in later life.[7] As people grow older, they tend to be more and more themselves. Their experience of many years has made them discard superficial imitations (common in youth) and has taught them what—to them—is important, and what is not. Self-esteem ("How do I feel about myself?") is another matter. The American culture is not marked by reverence for age; in fact, as we have seen, it glorifies youth. Among other influences, Americans are the result of a tremendous industrial development, and in handling new machines youth is an asset, and age is not. By and large, Americans fear old age, dislike thinking about it, and avoid those who personify it. This hardly produces a cheerful condition for the elderly, who recognize themselves that their eyes and ears are not as sharp as they used to be; that they are becoming forgetful; and that their physical prowess is decreasing. With the increasing number of senior citizens, accompanied by an increase in political power, the elderly may be less at a disadvantage. The nurse is in a good position to foster clients' self-esteem. Few people see much of the elderly without being struck by their ability to deal with their problems—some inevitable, some able to be improved: physical decline, loneliness, neglect, and above all, uselessness and the feeling of no longer being wanted or needed.

During older adulthood, very important and very difficult personal changes may take place. A man becomes a widower, a woman a widow. Retirement affects not only the formerly employed, but also their spouses. Men and women already grandparents may become great-grandparents. And not infrequently, older persons remarry.

The adjustment of marriage, great at any time, can be particularly difficult for the elderly, but it is one way in which they solve their characteristic problem, loneliness. There may often be an age difference; sometimes the man in a second marriage may be 15 or 20 years younger than the woman, or vice versa. For practical financial considerations, people in this age group sometimes live together without marrying. If a widow's inheritance is a trust fund that will end if she remarries, or if her social security will cease, marriage with a retired man on a limited income might be impossible. Older adults living together without marriage often face the disapproval of their grown children, friends, and neighbors; some solve this problem by moving to a new community, but the move in itself may create new problems, since it is less and less easy to make new friends as age increases. The nurse's role is to avoid being judgmental or moralistic. It is important for her to listen and to be interested in the possible effects such decisions will have on clients' health.

Late marriages, however, are often very successful. Factors contributing to success are a happy first marriage, knowledge of the traits to look for in a potential mate, marrying for love and a need for companionship rather than for convenience or money, similarity of education and social backgrounds, adequate incomes, approval of the marriage by children and friends, and reasonably good health.[5]

ENVIRONMENTAL CHANGES

This period also very frequently involves changes in living arrangements, which often have significant effects on health. This is one of the most radical personal changes of this age; it is necessitated by retirement with decreased income, by decreasing physical energy or perhaps some pathological condition, and most painfully, by the loss of a spouse. Since in this case the serious loss of a life companion is compounded by the serious loss of a familiar setting, it presents a particular danger to health.

VIGNETTE

Mrs. Miller was 72 years old when her husband died after a long illness. The couple had two children, a son and a daughter, both married, and both living in other states. Both invited their mother to make her home with them. She went to her son, who could give her a room of her own. But to reduce her furnishings to what one room could contain, she had to sell, give away, or take to the dump almost all her belongings. It was hard for her not to cry at the garage sale when she was offered fifty cents for the candy dish her husband gave her at their first Christmas. After 42 years of marriage, she moved away from her home and her friends to her son's house and all the adjustments that entailed.

Many older adults today have pleasant memories of living in a three-generation family where a grandfather or grandmother was responsible for giving them many happy childhood experiences. They tend to feel the best solution for them in their old age will be to move in with a son or daughter. In many cases, this can indeed be an excellent arrangement, but not always. These elderly adults sometimes do not realize the extent of the social changes in family life. Brought up themselves in the "children-should-be-seen-but-not-heard" school, they do not recognize what sweeping alterations "permissiveness" has brought, and how child-centered many homes are today. The elderly like peace and quiet; their grandchildren are rock fans. Few houses today are large enough to provide room and privacy for the differing generations. Though the nurse should not forget that plenty of grandparents today can be happy—and can give happiness—in their children's homes, still the odds have risen against this arrangement working out as well today as it did 70 years ago. The nurse may become involved in such decisions because often health crises occur at such times.

There is growing evidence that many older people not only wish to live apart from their children, but are happier and better off doing so.[8] Today, seven out of ten people over 65 maintain their own households. For elderly people who need financial help, some interest is beginning to develop in ways to make it possible for them to stay in their own homes rather than move to institutions, and this trend may continue. The nurse of course should be aware of such community programs as meals-on-wheels and home aides.

Money is perhaps the most important limitation on choice of living arrangements. Often, there is a regrettable reluctance to discuss money in the family circle. Some people feel this somehow cheapens family relationships. Nothing could be more unrealistic. The nurse should encourage clients to face financial situations frankly and openly, for in direct proportion to this openness is the chance of a successful outcome.

Some older adults, wanting to feel secure and settle money matters once and for all, turn over all their possessions to a family member or friend, in return for an oral or written guarantee of care and services for the rest of their lives. This is usually unwise. Many of us have heard of a mother who turned over her money to her daughter, moved in, was unhappy and complained, and then was told if she didn't like it to move out. It is wise to look for some arrangement less personal than living with, or entrusting one's financial resources to, one's family.

Some single men and women are so much a part of the families of a brother or sister that they fit in quite naturally. Others, however, are independent by nature, have plenty of interests and friends, and continue to live alone. Some persons want companionship and set up house with a friend or relative. Others may like to take on the position of housekeeper or companion for an invalid. In general, single adults enjoy their retirement in familiar surroundings near family, friends, and former coworkers. Older adults can move to new locations—particularly to milder climates—and start a new life; but it is wise to consider all the implications before taking an irrevocable step. Many have been disappointed; they find you can talk *to* the mountains or the ocean, but not *with* them.

A growing phenomenon is the building of retirement homes, and the nurse should be aware of this type of community facility. If Mrs. Miller had decided to enter one of these, she might have found some advantages over moving in with her son. She would have remained in her own community, in touch with her life-long friends; and her associates would be approximately her age and might share her interests. There would be none of the emotional strain that might develop if she did not care for the way her daughter-in-law was bringing up her grandchildren, and offered advice. If her presence in her son's home led to overcrowded conditions or constant friction about family behavior, the emotional strain might be particularly great.

The nurse can tell clients that none of them should assume that they will never need any of these substitute living arrangements for themselves or their parents; nor, on the other hand, should they assume that they will. At present, only about 5 percent of those over 65 live in this type of arrangement, although the percentage would undoubtedly be higher if more opportunities were available.

There is a critical need in our society for housing that can accommodate the special requirements of the elderly for independent living. At present, a variety of resources are available: residence halls, detached apartments, single homes, and multitype units. But they are few in number and in many communities none exist at all. In other communities some exist, but not enough to fill the need; they are filled and have long waiting lists. Some have restrictions on age and state of health. The nurse will help by suggesting thorough investigation of possibilities *before* a crisis arises. Clients are often reluctant to take this suggestion; as we have said, Americans in general tend to fear and dislike old age, and many find it hard or impossible to bring themselves to consider it until they are forced to do so. This feeling is understandable; but it is clear that for health and happiness it is necessary to prepare, within one's means, for the best living arrangements possible in old age.

DEVELOPMENTAL TASKS

For the older adult, there are four major developmental tasks with which the nurse can be of help.

The first is *recognizing that aging can be a positive experience.* This frequently involves a life review.[9-11] This can occur during the middle years too, but it is particularly important for the older adult. In general, men conduct a life review at the end of their career, and women when their children leave home.

The life review assists the elderly in putting their house in order, and it can enhance health by reducing and resolving conflict and strain. Some older adults are consciously aware of what they are doing; others are not. Some cannot bear to remember the pain of the past. Thus the intensity of the experience varies from mild and pleasant reminiscence to feverish preoccupation with a past particular event or subject. The contribution of the nurse as a listener is to try to shift emphasis from "What a mistake I made! How I wish I had done differently!" to "What did I learn from the experience which has made me better able to live my life fully?"

This tendency of the elderly to remember has sometimes been devalued and referred to as "living in the past," "second childhood," or "senility." It may be regarded somewhat more sympathetically as an expression of loneliness. It has been considered boring, time-consuming, and meaningless. Quite the contrary. It has a positive function, for in it older adults reflect on life in order to resolve, reorganize, and reintegrate what may be troubling or preoccupying them.[9]

Today, with the availability of the tape recorder, it is very easy to record material. Some people prefer to write down their memories, but many lack facility for doing that. Young and middle adults usually take little interest in family history; they are very busy, and they have little free time. But later in life they begin to think back. It is common to hear an older person say, "I wish I knew more about my grandparents! My mother's family came from Scotland (or Sweden or Russia). My grandfather fought in the Spanish-American War (or built the first schoolhouse in this county, or started such-and-such an industry in this state). When I was young, my grandmother sometimes wanted to tell me stories. I wasn't interested then, but now that I am, there's no one left of whom I can ask questions." Older adults who for their own sake are interested in finding out more about family history can be sure that eventually their descendants will be very grateful for any information they may leave. Visits to the place of birth, "the old home"; family, school, college, and church reunions; scrap books, photo albums, old letters, and memorabilia are rich sources of information. Many an elderly person engaged in this kind of activity develops interests to be pursued for the rest of life. According to Lewis and Butler, the most introspective part of life seems to occur in the sixties.[9]

Some schools are conducting programs where senior citizens who have had personal experience of a given period tell school children about it and answer their questions. In many cases, these programs have been very popular, and they serve the desirable function of bringing different generations together. If the nurse is aware of community projects of this sort, clients can be informed of them. In any case, the nurse can be an interested listener as to how clients are progressing in their own projects.

The second task is *making adjustments and redefining physical and social space.* Retirement is one example. "I married my husband for life but not for lunch," says one wife. "All he does all day long is tell me how I should clean house—which I've done for 40 years without his help," says another. Husband and wife must work out some means of meeting the situation. Household habits may require change with the development of physical disabilities. Arthritis may make it impossible to continue doing the laundry in the basement. Angina may make it necessary to move from a house to an apartment with elevator service. Since all of these changes require adjustment at a period when the capacity for adjustment is decreasing, the nurse can be of great help in giving advice based on physiological conditions as well as emotional ones. Often physical or economic reasons make this task crucial. All elderly adults, sooner or later, experience some changes which require some adjustment.

The third task is *to maintain feelings of self-worth, pride, and usefulness.* Emotional needs which have been met before now require new ways of fulfillment, and for many this task is not easy. Recreation often plays an important role here, but opportunities may be limited in many ways: physically, for example, by poor eyesight; economically, by a reduced income. (Incidentally, following the weather has been recommended as an ideal hobby for the elderly. It is free, it doesn't require eagle-eyed sight, and if in your vicinity there is nothing spectacular happening, somewhere there is some interesting weather always going on.) Education can be a factor. Reading requires little energy and gives much enjoyment. Most public libraries have a large selection of large-print books particularly for the elderly, and many librarians take great interest in advising elderly clients in finding books they will enjoy. Libraries also often have displays, frequently changed, which suggest new and interesting fields to explore. Those with limited education, however, may never have developed the habit of reading and find it too late to do so; they depend mainly on television for recreation. With all the criticism that television receives, it still remains true that at no period in history has there been available to so many such a wide variety of experiences; at no period in history has there been so good an opportunity for the elderly to broaden their world. Radio serves the same purpose for those with impaired eyesight.

In general, women cultivate a fairly wide range of recreational interests, many of which they carry throughout life. If it is necessary to give up fine embroidery, knitting may still be possible. Cooking can be continued, and with more leisure women may even bake their own bread. Cooking, incidentally, is not confined to women; many men living alone are excellent cooks. In general, however, men tend to limit their recreational interests to sports, and in this age range they can often only be spectators. Retirement complexes and homes for the aged are well provided with recreation suited to their residents. Those who live in their own homes or with children are not so well supplied, especially if their health is poor or transportation problems prevent them from participating in community-sponsored recreational activities. It is important for the nurse not to limit anticipatory guidance to purely physiological matters but also to supply information on what community opportunities exist, for these will ultimately have an important effect on health.

Companionship is very important for the successful completion of this task. To be of service to a friend contributes to the feeling of usefulness, and as friends grow older there may be increased opportunities of service. In many small towns or in city neighborhoods, one older adult man or woman may take over the function of "the driver," and transport friends who have given up their cars. Undeniably, there is a rather sad side to this topic: every year the circle of old friends narrows. Couples whose children went to school together and who in those days attended school games and functions together now find they have little in common when the children have grown up and gone away; someone moves away; someone dies. And retired person do not meet new friends in the course of business, as formerly they were constantly doing.

But there are ways of making new friends at this age, too, and the nurse, mindful that this is an important problem, should be alert for opportunities in the community to recommend. The school project is one example. Practically everywhere today there are senior citizen groups, which offer a great variety of activities, celebrate members' birthdays, include a "sunshine committee" who call on members in hospitals, and so on. Calling on a friend in a nursing home may result in meeting other people there. Shut-ins are very grateful for visits or notes. A great advantage of attending a church (in addition to the religious aspect, of which we shall be speaking) is that there the elderly have opportunities for contact with middle and young adults; lack of this contact is a disadvantage in communities planned purely for the elderly.

Occasionally, an elderly woman or man living alone whose relatives live far away is adopted as "grandmother" or "grandfather" by a young couple with small children moving into the neighborhood because their blood relatives also are far away. Such an older man or woman may have time to show the children special skills, such as patchwork quilting or cabinet work, that their parents have not time or expertise for. Elder persons possessing such skills are very valuable as consultants for groups like Brownies or Scouts. Contract bridge requires four players; a man or woman available to make a fourth may be in great demand and may meet new friends that way. The nurse can collect as many suggestions as possible from clients, so that at Christmas, looking through the address book, clients may balance the names crossed off of old friends lost during the year with the names of new friends gained.

The last developmental task is to *strive toward developing a personal set of goals as one prepares for death*. At this time it is normal for interest to shift from others to oneself; it helps adults accept the inevitability of death and prepare for this goal before it comes. There may be increased interest in religion, which is valuable far beyond the social companionship, to which we have referred. It fosters thought about the greatest mystery of life; death.

Elderly adults today, according to Hurlock, commonly ask three questions.[5] The first is "When will I die?" This, of course, cannot be answered. Still, they think about it; they wish to complete "unfinished business." The second is "What is likely to cause my death?" Again, this cannot be answered, but it preoccupies people at this age. Whenever possible, the nurse should do as much as possible to allay any unwarranted fears it rouses. "Will it be a long-term illness? Will it bankrupt me? Will my last days be painful?" While none of these questions have definite answers, the nurse is in a position at least to dissipate superstitions and unnecessary fears.

And thirdly, "How can I die as I wish to die?" Today, with the great strides of modern medicine in prolonging life, many older adults fear prolongation of life more than death. They believe they have a right to determine their manner of death, to be spared a long debilitating illness, and to die in dignity and peace. This is a highly controversial question, with far too many ramifications to be entered into here; but two statements can be made. First, the nurse should not try to prevent clients from discussing this question. On the contrary, they should be encouraged to pursue it fully and freely. Second, they should be encouraged to discuss it with their physician. If they find that he or she does not agree with them, they can be advised to consider finding a physician who does, while it is still in their power to do so.

The mystery of death—still the greatest of all human mysteries, still unsolved in spite of various answers which bring great sureness and comfort to many—is a subject the nurse must not evade. Many families cannot bear to talk about dying with their old members, and even some health care personnel are reluctant to do so because they feel they do not have answers to give. But it is important that older adults should not only think about it themselves, but be able to discuss it with someone else. Death is the end of life as we know it here; it is also a part of life and an impending certainty for the very elderly.

In assessing and providing anticipatory guidance to older adults as they accomplish these four tasks, perhaps the most important thing the nurse can do is to encourage them to use these years to grow. Lewis and Butler, in reference to the life review, stated that

The success of the life review depends on the outcomes of the struggle to resolve old issues of resentment, guilt, bitterness, mistrust, dependence and nihilism. All of the truly significant emotional options remain available until the moment of death—love, hate, reconciliation, self-assertion, and self-esteem.[9]

The nurse can help clients realize that their lives have potential for self-actualization and the enrichment of others until the moment of death.

BIBLIOGRAPHY

1* Butler, Robert N., and Myrna I. Lewis: *Aging and Mental Health*, The C. V. Mosby Company, St. Louis, 1973.

2* Lamy, Peter P.: "Aging: How Human Physiology Responds," in Ewald Busse (ed.), *Theory and Therapeutics of Aging*, Medcome, New York, 1973.

3* Kennedy, Robert H.: "Easing Into Old Age," *Bull. New York Acad. Med.* 47: 1432–1439, 1971.

4 Blum, J. E., L. L. Fosshage, and L. F. Javvik: "Intellectual Changes and Sex Differences in Octogenarians: A Twenty-Five Year Longitudinal Study of Aging," *Developmental Psych.* 7: 178–187, 1972.

5 Hurlock, Elizabeth B.: *Developmental Psychology*, 4th ed., McGraw-Hill Book Company, New York, 1975.

6 Neugarten, B. L.: "Grow Old With Me: The Best is Yet to Be," *Psychol. Today*, 5: 45–46, 1971.

7 Atchley, Robert C.: *The Social Forces in Later Life*, Wadsworth Publishing Company, Inc., Belmont, Calif., 1972.

8 Randall, Ollie A.: *Family, Friends and Living Arrangements*, rev. ed., Industrial Relations Center, The University of Chicago, Chicago, 1966.

9* Lewis, Myrna I., and Robert N. Butler: "Life-Review Therapy—Putting Memories to Work in Individual and Group Psychotherapy," *Geriatrics*, November 1974, pp. 165–173.

10 Kastenbaum, Robert: ". . . Gone Tomorrow," *Geriatrics*, November 1974, pp. 127–134.

11 Weinburg, Jack: "What Do I Say to My Mother When I Have Nothing to Say?" *Geriatrics*, November 1974, pp. 155–159.

12* Brantl, Virginia M., and Sister Marie Raymond Brown (eds.): *Readings in Gerontology*, The C. V. Mosby Company, St. Louis, 1973.

*Starred items are of particular interest.

CHAPTER 12

Activity, Rest, and Safety

EXERCISE

While no one would claim that a person at the age of 75 can be as physically active as one at age 45, without question the majority of our older adults get less exercise than they could profit from. According to the National Adult Physical Fitness Survey, only 39 percent of Americans age 60 and over get any systematic exercise. Their favorite form of exercise is walking, practiced by 46 percent of the men and 33 percent of the women. Few indulge in anything more strenuous: 1 percent jog, 6 percent do calisthenics, 3 percent ride bicycles, and 4 percent swim. Yet 71 percent of them believe they get all the exercise they need.[1] According to C. Carson Conrad, Executive Director of the President's Council on Physical Fitness and Sports, this misconception arises because older persons believe their need for exercise diminishes with increasing age and eventually disappears; they greatly exaggerate the risks of vigorous exercise after middle age; they overrate the benefits of light and sporadic exercise; and they underrate their own abilities and capacities.[1]

It is well established that a regular program of exercise slows the aging process, as well as those degenerative diseases associated with aging. In extreme old age, there comes a time when exercise beyond that of the simplest acts of living becomes impossible; but this day can be almost indefinitely postponed. The age of retirement is no time to take it easy, but to stay active.

Benefits of Exercise Psychologically, exercise is beneficial. It induces relaxation; serves as a release for nervous tension, strain, and anxiety; and helps to provide restful sleep. And the physiological benefits of exercise are numerous.

Exercise establishes or maintains the general tone throughout the body, including that of the heart muscle itself. It also keeps in good tone the diaphragm, another very important muscle (as do deep breathing programs). Good muscle tone is important, since the muscles throughout the body help the blood flow to and from the heart. It is the pumping action of the diaphragm which helps the suction of the blood back to the chambers of the right side of the heart. Exercise is of great benefit to the digestion of food and in reducing nervous tension, which is a common factor in cases of esophageal irritability (cardiospasm) and peptic ulcer. Also, it has a favorable effect on bowel function. Moreover, since it helps to control the appetite and burn off extra calories, it helps to control obesity (a benefit at any age).

Finally, the deepening of respiration which exercise produces enhances the function of the lungs in gaseous exchange and the state of the lung tissue itself. Although chronic bronchitis and emphysema are common in old age and do limit the amount of exercise possible, they do not rule out *all* exercise. Many patients with heart disease are benefited by suitable exercise. Of course, angina pectoris too easily induced or myocardial weakness of considerable degree will demand absolute rest pro tem, but with recovery, or in the presence of well-healed myocardial infarctions, a careful program may not only be an important health measure but may even retard the further progress of coronary atherosclerosis.

The nurse should remember that each client must be individually considered. While exercise in general is desirable, no program should even be considered before the client has had a physical examination and his doctor has evaluated what limitations on activity may exist. Two special conditions are relevant at this age: a sense of balance and muscular flexibility. The nurse may suggest special exercise to improve these if necessary. Older adults, particularly if they wear bifocals or trifocals, are much happier and more independent with a good sense of balance, which can enable them to go up and down stairs frequently and use public transportation. The greater the degree of muscular flexibility in the older adult, the greater the self-reliance. To be able to do things for yourself is a financial advantage, and an even greater psychological one.

Beginning an Exercise Program In "The Fitness Challenge . . . in the Later Years," which the nurse can recommend to clients, the Administration on Aging has developed three programs of exercise, each with a pre-exercise test and careful instructions as to starting positions, actions, order, and precautions. Exercises include, among others, the walk, the alternate walk-jog, bending and stretching, rotating the head, raising the legs, walking a straight line, knee push-ups, and the stork stand.[2]

Clients who have been particularly inactive might be encouraged to begin gradually by first walking more in daily living: getting up to get a glass of water during TV commercials; walking around the table or up and down the hall; and in good weather walking outside to the mail box, to the store, or to see a friend. Walking is an excellent exercise for many older adults, but for best results it should be brisk, regular, and sustained, and clients can be encouraged to progress to this stage.

Dancing is another good exercise, particularly for those who have been accustomed to ballroom dancing. Clients unfamiliar with this form might enjoy folk dancing. Swimming is another excellent way to exercise: moving the arms under water, walking or marching in water up over the knees, or floating on the stomach or back with a flutter kick. Many older adults have not had the experience of physical education classes, and to them the nurse may suggest resources at the local YMCA, YWCA, or Red Cross where they may learn new sports.

Many older adults enjoy exercising together. The National Association for Human Development has completed "Join the Active People Over 60," a pilot workshop designed to encourage the growth of physical fitness and health education programs for the nation's elderly.[1,3] Many senior citizen centers are instituting exercise and physical fitness programs, with activities such as swimming, bowling, golf, horseshoes, ping pong, and boccie.

But it is always to be remembered that this is not the age for competition. Senior citizens should compete only with themselves and should have programs custom-made for their own individual needs.

There are some interesting statistics which the nurse should remember. A recent study of 268 persons aged 60 to 94, carried on over a period of 11 years, showed that of the three health-related practices examined—inactivity, obesity, and cigarette smoking—inactivity had the highest correlation with illness indicators. The number of those who spent 2 or more weeks in bed per year was 2½ times greater among those with fewer locomotor activities, the number of those who received three or more physician's visits per year 1½ times greater. In the group with few locomotor activities, one-half died sooner than actuarily expected, compared to between one-fourth and one-third of the others.[4] Clearly, then, exercise is of imperative importance for maintenance and promotion of health in the older adult.

It is not necessary to limit the encouragement of exercise merely to physical fitness programs. The nurse who encourages older clients to get involved in a range of activities, such as paid employment, volunteer work, care of the home and garden, travel, and hobbies, will be fostering exercise as a bonus in addition to the other benefits these interests will bestow.

SLEEP

Though older adults may not sleep as many hours as they did formerly, rest is very important for them. Sensible rest periods and sensible pacing are necessary to provide the energy for a full life.

Old age normally brings with it a decline in the amount of sleep. Compared to the sleep pattern of the young adult, the older adult has a disrupted sleep pattern with more awakenings, less and more disordered REM sleep, and decrease in stage 4 sleep. The disordered REM mechanism might be reflected in either or both the ability to recall dreams and the content of dreams.[5] In studies, older adults report dream recall from REM awakening of 43.5 percent as compared to 87 percent in young adult population.[6] Thus by the age of 60 or 70, persons usually need an hour or two less than before, and the sleep itself is no longer the unbroken sleep of the young adult but alternates resting or wakefulness with sleep. Long-term or unusual sleep problems should of course be referred to a physician, but older adults should recognize that changes in their sleep patterns are to be expected, and that most old people will face some degree of insomnia, especially women.

Older adults are prone to turn to drugs to help them sleep. This is not the answer. Depressant drugs actually tend to reduce the amount of deep sleep (and deep sleep is necessary for health) and may even become addicting. For simple insomnia, the nurse can recommend such things as reading in the middle of the night until drowsiness returns. Many older adults get great comfort from a small bedside radio, and they find it interesting to pick up programs from far-off stations which they cannot get when the air channels are crowded during the day. For others, this may be a good time to go back to poetry, memorized long ago and now recalled with deeper meanings given by life experience. It may be a good time to recall vacations and trips of all sorts, interesting places visited, and little adventures encountered, and to relive pleasant memories of the past.

Though older adults sleep less at night, they become increasingly prone to napping during the day, a very useful practice which provides rest and relaxation. Since, by and large, the older adult group are retired persons, the plan of their days is under their own control, and there is no reason why they should not nap whenever they feel like it. A little extra sleep during the day is very good compensation for less sleep during the night.

SAFETY

Older adults are at special risk for safety. It is particularly important for the nurse to encourage them to take precautions and establish certain habits. Falls are a particular problem. Healing occurs more slowly in direct proportion to advancing age, and there also may be decreased bone density, so that the seriousness of a fall is greatly enhanced at this time. Many accidents occur to older persons at night; they wake up, feel confused, perhaps are partially medicated, get up, and fall. The nurse can emphasize that a flashlight by the bed is indispensable, as is forming the habit of always turning it on; and that it is very unwise to move bedroom furniture around into new positions. A list of safety precautions for the older adult does not differ in kind from a list of safety precautions for anyone else; but it is just more important that the older adult follow them scrupulously.

In the house, handrails should be provided for all stairways, including the one to the basement. A householder may have walked up and down those stairs for 50 years without falling; never mind, put a handrail in *now*. Stairs should be kept clear of all objects and should be well lighted, and top and bottom steps should be painted white (or given some obvious identification). Passageways should be well lighted at night, particularly that between bedroom and bathroom. Throw rugs should be tacked down or fitted with no-slip pads. No electric light cords should trail across the floor. Light switches should be well located, that is, at the head of the bed and the top and bottom of stairs, and older adults should form a firm habit of always turning on lights and never groping about in the dark. Again, a bedside flashlight is indispensable.

In the kitchen, a small step ladder or stool should be sturdy and be put securely in place before use. Ideally, an older adult should never use one unless someone else is at hand. Women should wear shoes with good broad heels; laced shoes should always be securely tried. The danger of slipping is great in the kitchen, where the floor is usually waxed, and any water spilled should be wiped up immediately. In winter when snow is often tracked in, this precaution is especially important.

In the bathroom, the temperature of shower or tub should

always be checked before entering the water. There should be a rubber mat in the tub, and a firm grab bar fixed to the wall. An elderly person gets out of a tub more safely from a kneeling than from a sitting position: that is, getting to the knees and facing the back of the tub, taking firm hold of the bar in the wall with one hand, and then stepping over the edge of the tub.

In any room, a new arrangement of furniture is a hazard.

Many older adults take medications, and their safe use calls for a list of do's and don'ts. Do throw away outdated medications. Do pour a liquid medication from the unlabeled side of the bottle so that the label can be seen. If two medications look alike, do put a special mark on each to distinguish them. Do learn the names of drugs, their side effects, and how they look. Do call your pharmacist or doctor immediately if a refill of a prescription looks different from the original; it may be the same medication from a different company, but it may be a mistake. Do check. Do keep a current list of all the medications you are taking and take it with you to all your doctors, dentist, and eye doctor.

Don't take any medication in the dark; always turn the light on. Don't mix several kinds of pills in one box; keep them separate. Don't keep cleaning liquids in the medicine cabinet. And if medication is kept at the bedside, don't keep more than one night's supply there at a time.

Finally, driving a car presents a special safety hazard for elderly adults (not to mention their passengers). Older adults should take all safety precautions that any driver of any age should take (seeing that the car is always in good condition, following highway rules and safety maxims, planning long trips to avoid fatigue, and so on); but there is need for special care in this period. Vision and hearing problems begin to arise in middle age and now increase. The nurse should emphasize the importance of periodic checkups to make sure clients have the vision, hearing, and muscular coordination necessary to be safe drivers. Even if they are competent themselves, the nurse may well suggest they would be wise to avoid night driving; too many night drivers have had "one for the road," and visibility, of course, is less.

Fatigue has been found to be a special problem for the older adult. The nurse should advise clients to drive with companions to share the driving, and to take plenty of rest stops. It is better to get gas, walk around a bit, and then drive on before getting out to have a cup of coffee than to make one stop serve two purposes.

Older drivers, if they are retired persons, as is generally the case, can—and should—plan to drive at the less crowded times: weekdays rather than weekends, mid-morning and afternoon rather than rush hours. And they can allow plenty of time for back roads rather than take crowded highways. As they have the time, so they should have developed the judgment to "take it easy" and not over-tax themselves.

But there seems to be one special problem for older drivers: the tendency to go slow—*too* slow. On a turnpike the slow driver is a real safety hazard and the cause of many accidents. Drivers at the legal limit cannot adapt themselves to the snail's pace, grow im-patient, want to pass, and pull out into oncoming traffic. No one wants older drivers to speed; but if they find themselves uncom-fortable doing 50 or 55 miles per hour on the highway, this is a definite warning that they should not be driving there, and this warning should not be ignored.

The importance of the automobile in American life is a phe-nomenon truly to be wondered at. For the teenager, getting the driver's license is a significant mark of maturity; it may even seem more important than casting the first vote. For many older persons, the car seems to be a symbol of independence to which they cling tenaciously. Younger persons find it hard to comprehend how sensitive an area this is. The nurse, aware of psychological as well as physiological factors, can bring up the topic with clients over several visits or over several years; safety is always an eligible topic to discuss. With increasing age, the stakes of car injury and danger, not only to the driver but also to others, become higher and higher.

BIBLIOGRAPHY
1* Conrad, C. Carson: "When You're Young at Heart," *Aging*, April 1976, pp. 11–13.
2* *The Fitness Challenge. . .in the Later Years*, Superintendent of Documents Distribution Center, Pueblo, Colo. 81009, 116C, 1973.
3 "Workshops Spark Fitness Programs," *Aging*, April 1976, pp. 14–17.
4 Palmore, Erdman (Ed.): "Normal Aging. II. Reports from the Duke Longitudinal Studies, 1970–1973," Duke University Press, Durham, N.C., 1974.
5 Kramer, Milton, Thomas Roth, and John Trinder: "Dreams and Dementia: A Laboratory Exploration of Dream Recall and Dream Content in Chronic Brain Syndrome," *Internat. J. Aging Human Development*, vol. 6 (2), Boywood Publishing Co., 1975, pp. 172–182.
6 Kahn, E., C. Fisher, and L. Lieberman: "Dream Recall in the Normal Aged," *Amer. Geriat. Soc.*, 17: 1121–1126, 1969.
7 Bortz, Edward L.: *Better Health After Fifty*, pp. 72–73, The Retirement Council, New York, 1964.
8* Cooper, Kenneth H.: *The New Aerobics*, Bantam Books, Inc., New York, 1970.

9* Sussman, A., and R. Goode: *The Magic of Walking*, Simon & Schuster, Inc., New York, 1967.

10* Jonas, D. G., and D. J. Jonas: *Young Til We Die*, Coward, McCann & Geoghegan, Inc., New York, 1973.

11* Winter, R.: *Ageless Aging: How to Extend Your Healthy and Productive Years*, Crown Publishers, Inc., New York, 1973.

*Starred items are of special interest.

CHAPTER 13

Nutrition and the Older Adult

According to our evidence, in general, American older adults do not eat well, nor do they eat as well as they might. "No population group in America, among the middle classes, eats so poorly as do the men and women in the later years of life,"[1] according to Deutsch. Generally speaking, malnutrition in the United States is not due to lack of foodstuffs of appropriate quality or quantity. And though lack of money may be a contributing factor in poor nutrition for the elderly, many who could be called rich eat worse than their contemporaries who are poor. One study of persons over 60 years of age showed evidence of general undernutrition that was not restricted to the very poor or to any single ethnic group. Poor food choices and poor use of money available for food were significant factors.

THE OLDER ADULT DIET

Caloric requirements decrease with age, due to a lower basal metabolism, decreased cell mass, and decreased activity. In general, the reduction in caloric need is approximately −7.5 percent for each decade past 25 years of age. For the older adult woman, the average recommended calorie requirement is 1800; for the older adult man, 2000. However, calorie requirements are highly individual and must be calculated according to personal factors.

Many clients think that after retirement the body's nutrient needs diminish because of the slowdown of body processes. They are mistaken. A comparison of key recommended allowances at ages 35 and 75 shows that those for protein, vitamins A, D, E, C, B_2, B_6, and B_{12}, folacin, calcium, phosphorus, and magnesium have not declined in the slightest. For men, iron needs remain the same, though it decreases for women when menstruation ceases. Niacin needs stay the same for women, but go down slightly for men, as do thiamine needs. The nurse, then, must discuss with clients ways to include all these essentials in a diet of fewer calories.[1, 2]

For older adults, nutrition is an environmental factor under their own control; by proper nutrition, they can help themselves to prevent disease and disability, and to recover from illness and accidental injury.[3, 4] We already know a good deal about diet and the degenerative diseases and about how good diet can prevent them; good diet may also have some effect in retarding the aging process. There is some evidence that while osteoporosis does not seem to be reversed by high-calcium diets, the need for calcium in old age does not decrease. Iron is required in at least normal amounts, and there is some evidence that if fluoride is consumed throughout life, it may decrease osteoporosis.

In reducing calories, crash diets are to be avoided since they may lack essential nutrients. Weight reduction should be gradual. For elderly obese or overweight, it is important to lose weight; and cutting down on excessive saturated fats and cholesterol is an excellent way to also slow down the progress of arteriosclerosis. Another desirable reduction is that of excessive consumption of sugar, often prevalent in the older adult diet (as indeed in the general diet). This is important not only because it helps reduce total daily calories, but also because it reduces obesity and may avoid the development of diabetes mellitus. It is certainly conducive to better dental health. A good way for the older adult to reduce calories is to eat less food more often. If older persons eat small meals frequently, they are less likely to be truly hungry and therefore to overindulge. Some good practices to follow are eating smaller portions of all foods; eating less fat; eating fewer fried foods; trimming excess fat off meat; using low-fat milk; substituting fruit for rich pastries and sweets; and including adequate fruits, vegetables, and whole grain breads or cereals. Roughage is a diet essential, best provided by cereal, bran, and vegetables. Plenty of water should be drunk. Excessive consumption of salt is to be avoided in order to prevent excessive fluid retention and elevation of blood pressure. This can be a particular problem for older people, since they tend to eat a good many canned, frozen, or convenience foods (all highly salted) and frequently eat out in restaurants.

Jean Mayer, Professor of Nutrition at Harvard University, points out three areas in which nutrition is of importance in aging.[5] First, through such factors as decreased income, increasing disabilities, and loneliness, aging interferes with good nutrition. Second, nutrition is involved with the development of many diseases associated with old age. Third, the relationship of nutrition to the normal aging process needs further study. Diet in old age, then, may have much more importance than is generally realized.

When counseling older adults, the nurse should be aware that the recommended daily dietary allowances (RDDA or RDA) developed by the Food and Nutrition Board of the National Academy of Sciences, are defined as "allowances intended to serve as goals for planning food supplies and as guides for interpretation of the food consumption of all groups of people."[6] However, since these were designed for a typical healthy man of 25, the nurse should use them only as a "guide" in dealing with elderly clients.

Donald Deutsch, in *The Family Guide to Better Food and Better Health*, gives a rule of thumb for the older adult's daily diet: "One or two glasses of milk (preferably skim or low-fat); at least one large serving of meat, fish, or poultry; at least one serving of green or yellow vegetables; one or two servings of citrus fruit or tomatoes; possibly a serving of other vegetables such as potatoes; two or three servings of bread, flour, or cereals; and one or two tablespoons of table fat (such as margarine)."[1] Water is also very important, since often the older adult does not drink enough liquids. Three to five cups a day should be a minimal requirement.

DIET DEFICIENCIES AND MODIFICATIONS

That these ideal norms are not generally met is evidenced by various studies. According to one, older adults have significant dietary deficiencies as determined by the USDA average data: for men, 21 to 29 percent omission of calcium, 1 to 10 percent deficit of vitamin A and vitamin C, and an 11 to 20 percent deficit of riboflavin; for women, over 30 percent deficiency of calcium, 1 to 10 percent deficits in iron and vitamin A, 11 to 20 percent deficit of riboflavin and thiamine. "Over 75, the dietary deficiencies of vitamin A and riboflavin increase markedly."[1]

According to the Ten State Nutrition Survey (1968–1970), undernutrition in persons over 60 years of age was not limited to the very poor or to any single ethnic group.[7] The deficiencies were due to poor food choices, resulting inadequate diets, and poor use of money available for food, particularly neglect of foods rich in vitamin A and of excellent, low-cost sources of protein. Low vitamin C levels were more prevalent in men than in women and increased with age. Iron seemed to be the greatest problem in all ethnic groups and income levels, but especially among low-income blacks. Riboflavin was a problem in blacks at both high and low income levels and in Spanish-Americans at low income levels, as was vitamin A. Thiamine did not appear to be deficient.

Decreased vitamin intake may be due to a variety of reasons: physiological, social, or economic. Some diseases may reduce the absorption of vitamins. A deficiency in vitamin B is sometimes responsible for the mental confusion often observed in old people, and this may lead to a vicious cycle, the confusion causing lack of desire to eat and the resulting inadequate diet causing more confusion. Deficiencies in the fat-soluble vitamins A, D, and E are frequently due to a low-fat diet (tea and toast), or to interference in absorption caused by habitual ingestion of mineral oil as a laxative.

In spite of the deficiencies observed in the diets of older adults, nutritional supplements such as vitamin pills are not necessary if the diet is adequate and well balanced. However, according to Krehl, "the use of a regular supplement or at least a maintenance level of required vitamins and minerals is reasonable nutritional insurance and may be provided at low cost."[8] But it is difficult to demonstrate that megavitamins achieve any type of supernutritional status. In fact, an excess of the water-soluble vitamins is usually excreted in the urine. An excess of fat-soluble vitamins, particularly vitamins A and D at high-dosage levels, is actually dangerous and should be prohibited.

There may be a special need in the older adult diet for more vitamin E. Vitamin E is not one vitamin, but a group; one of its functions is to protect the lipids that construct the cell wall. In aging, the gradual diminishing of cells may be in part due to deterioration of the lipids that make up a large part of their wall structure.[2, 9] Some authorities recommend supplemental vitamin E and question whether the RDDA of 30 IU of vitamin E is sufficient for the older adult.

However, many older adults are prime targets for fad and supplement promoters. These supplements are often expensive, and in many cases the money might better be spent on foods containing the vitamins in natural form. Good food sources of vitamin E are vegetable oils, wheat germ, milk, eggs, muscle meats, fish, cereals, and leafy vegetables. Vitamin E, as well as all the other vitamins and minerals, must not be overlooked in diet planning for, and by, older adults.

In this age range, tooth and gum problems may require some diet modifications. According to one study,[7] the prevalance of periodontal disease increased with age to over 90 percent in nearly every subgroup of the people surveyed at the age range from 65 to 74. It was more prevalent in men than in women. The percentage of edentulous persons also increased with age and was highest among whites, reaching 55 percent at the age group 55 to 64.

Difficulty in chewing may thus result in a diet high in sugar and carbohydrates and low in protein. Dental attention is of course called for. Preparation of such foods as soups, stews, and casseroles, and grinding or chopping raw vegetables may reduce the problem. Fish, cottage cheese, yogurt, peanut butter, baked beans, eggs, ground meat, and poultry are all rich in protein; and all are comparatively soft, and therefore suitable for those who have difficulty in chewing.

Also in old age there may be a gradual diminution of the senses of taste and smell, which may result in loss of appetite. Variety is the cure for this: variety in flavor, texture, temperature, and appearance of food. An idea exists that spicy foods are bad for the older adult; this is a myth. True, some specific digestive disorders require bland diets; but for the ordinary older adult, spicy, highly flavored foods are entirely harmless and may revive a flagging appetite. To deal with loss of appetite, it is advisable to prepare small portions so that the eater does not feel overwhelmed, and to enrich the diet by fortifying milk drinks with eggs or ice cream and using whole milk instead of skim if gaining weight is not a problem. Another factor which sometimes causes difficulty is eating is mucosal changes in the mouth and a decrease in the quality of salivary secretions.

Constipation is a common problem among older adults; it may be caused by inactivity, decreased fluid intake, weak abdominal muscles, or a combination of these and other factors. It can be helped by a diet high in fluids and roughage (fresh and stewed fruits, particularly grandmother's time-honored prune juice, and plenty of salads and leafy vegetables) and moderate exercise.

When discussing diet with older adults, the nurse should not overlook any of these physical factors. However, personal factors in this field are of equal importance.

PSYCHOSOCIAL FACTORS

Poor eating habits may have many causes, among which are psychological and sociological factors. Clients may be poorly informed on basic nutrition; they may be guided by whim ("I just can't drink milk"; "Even as a child, I never could stand brocoli"); they may eat at odd times; they may spoil their appetite and their teeth by eating chocolates all day long. But they may also be severely handicapped by the conditions under which they live.

The nurse should investigate five areas, of which the first is cooking facilities. This is so important that a home visit may perhaps be necessary.

Some older adults do not have any cooking facilities at all and must therefore eat out. It is as important for them to be aware of their nutritional needs as for any people who do their own cooking. If money is a problem, it may be economical for them to take the main meal of the day in a restaurant, since nutritious breakfasts and lunches can be eaten with foods that require neither cooking nor refrigeration; dried milk, fresh fruits, breads and crackers, peanut butter, cheese, luncheon meats, and prepared cereals can form the basis for well-balanced meals. In this case, if they check the food guide given in Chapter 18 to see what they have already eaten that day before they go to dinner, they can secure the foods that remain. Even institutionalized adults, who eat meals prepared by others, would do well to assess their daily diet and supplement it, if necessary, with an extra glass of milk or piece of fruit.

The client may not have a stove. The nurse can suggest a hot plate, which will at once extend the range of food preparation. A double boiler also enlarges the range of the hot plate, for beans can be boiled in the bottom, for example, while rolls or canned meat are being warmed in the top.

The client may not have a refrigerator. The nurse can suggest buying an inexpensive Styrofoam cooler (of the sort often used on camping trips) and keeping it stocked with ice, which can be bought at a food store or from an outdoor dispenser. If the client does have a refrigerator, perhaps he or she is not making economical use of the freezing compartment. It is more economical to buy larger portions, and if this is done and several servings of a dish prepared at one time, all but the first can be frozen for a later day. Without a refrigerator, leftovers are a real problem. Many foods, such as tuna, canned vegetables, and canned baked beans, can be eaten at room temperature, but without refrigeration any leftovers from them should be thrown away because of the danger of spoilage. Many older adults can not afford to throw away leftovers, and the Styrofoam cooler would not only pay for itself in a short time but improve the quality and safety of meals.

The second area for the nurse to investigate for clients is transportation. Many adults whose cooking facilities are adequate to their needs are handicapped by lack of transportation: to markets, to food stamp centers, to group feeding programs. Shopping can be a real problem to an older adult who lives alone, in an isolated area, who may find it hard to get around freely because of a physical disability such as arthritis. In many places public transportation is inadequate, and taxis are expensive.

Axel is a bachelor, 76 years old, living in a third floor apartment in a building with no elevator. He has been retired for over 10 years. Walking up and down stairs becomes increasingly more difficult. When his legs were better, he used to go out frequently to shop and he did a good deal of cooking for himself, but he is now forced to rely mainly on canned goods. His real problem is shopping. For a number of years he patronized a neighborhood store which carried fresh meats and vegetables and fruits and would deliver; but it has recently closed down. Now he is reduced to eating what he can carry back himself from one monthly taxi trip to a supermarket—he cannot afford to go more often.

Axel's neighborhood store was typical of many, which are often patronized by older adults whose limited transportation forces them to shop within walking distance. These stores are usually more expensive than supermarkets and have a smaller selection of goods. The nurse should not necessarily advise clients not to use them, however, for many elderly persons prefer to shop there. The owner will know all the regular customers, and they will get to know each other; there may perhaps be a language bond if the client speaks a language other than English. Shopping there becomes a social affair; you are not hurried or made to feel guilty if the check-out clerk has to stop to weigh one or two potatoes for you, as you might at a supermarket where customers get theirs in 10 pound bags. Also, credit is usually easily available if needed. Shopping for food is not a matter of economy alone, but affects the clients' daily life and their enjoyment of it.

As the number of senior citizens increase, in many communities resources available to them are also increasing, and the nurse should be able to give clients information about them. "Meals-on-wheels" has become a familiar phrase. Some cities are inaugurating group feeding programs for senior citizens, utilizing school cafeterias when the school children are not using them. These meals are generally inexpensive, and many of the programs provide transportation to the centers. Other communities are initiating groups of home health aides, volunteers who will help elderly adults with shopping and sometimes even with meal preparations.

The third area for the nurse to consider is loneliness. Many older adults are lonely, and though this may be destructive in many ways, it has an obvious impact upon nutrition. As long as you prepare a meal for someone else, you give thought to good food, strive to serve it attractively, and therefore foster good nutrition for both eaters. If you are alone, why bother? It's easier to open a can of anything handy and eat it standing at the kitchen sink.

The nurse can make many suggestions here. To pack a lunch and eat it on the porch or in the park on a nice day will make a pleasant occasion. To set up a place mat in the dining room, or on a light movable table in the living room, will get you away from the kitchen sink! You can decorate it with a little plant or a flower or two; you can even grow your own, for a grapefruit or orange seed will develop into a charming little tree, and the sliced-off tops of carrots, in a shallow dish of water, will send up delicate fronds which will provide a attractive centerpiece for a number of weeks. A book, a magazine, or a favorite radio or TV program while you eat will banish the sense of isolation and produce a pleasant atmosphere for your meal. Moreover, a meal makes a fine opportunity for establishing contact with someone else who lives alone. Ask in a friend whom you may have met at a community program; the next step will be accepting a return invitation; and this may lead to regular interchanges in which each host or hostess enjoys finding something new and delicious for the guest. On a larger scale, senior citizen groups often stage potluck dinners.

The fourth area of concern is the serious one of alcohol and drug abuse. Both of these are highly destructive and may result in damage to the client's health because these clients often fail to eat a proper diet and develop malnutrition. It is in this period that a client who has drunk heavily over a number of years may show the effects. Also, due to senescence or disease, or both, the elderly exhibit a reduced drug tolerance.[10] Thus such drugs as the salicylates (aspirin) can cause vitamin K deficiency and damage the kidneys. Certain laxatives, including some available without prescription, can produce liver damage. In this age group, many clients are receiving multiple drug therapy from their physicians; some may be taking as many as ten or twelve different drugs. As people grow older, their response to drug treatment becomes more divergent. Therefore it is very important for the nurse to warn clients of the dangers of medication on their nutritional state, particularly over-the-counter medications.

Finally, the nurse must consider two kinds of limitations. The first is physical: with aging, the olfactory organs atrophy, with a resulting loss of smell and taste. This may lead to a very monotonous diet, since "everything tastes the same anyway," and the secret of a good diet is variety. Difficulty in chewing and swallowing may also contribute to a diet monotonous in texture and consistency if the older adult finds it too much trouble to bother with anything but canned soup and canned pears.

The second limitation, and a very common one in this age group, is financial. Many older adults live on a fixed income, and in our present inflationary spiral they find it very difficult to buy the foods they should have. Protein foods are among the most expensive, and so are fresh fruits and vegetables. As income shrinks, the buyer turns to items which are inexpensive and offer plenty of bulk, such as bread, rice, and spaghetti. But a diet over-balanced with starches will make the eater feel weak, lethargic, and continuously less inclined to make the effort required to eat better and secure the energy-producing proteins, vitamins, and minerals.

Here the nurse can make many suggestions. Cottage cheese is an excellent as well as a relatively inexpensive source of protein, as are eggs (incidentally, since the color of the eggshell does not affect the nutritional value of the egg, buy brown ones if they are cheaper than white ones). Textured vegetable proteins are now on the market which can be used as meat substitutes or extenders. Powdered milk is an excellent and inexpensive source of protein, and it can be added to a great variety of foods.

If it is feasible to have a small vegetable garden, elderly adults will not only relish their own fresh string beans and tomatoes but they will be in better health as a result of their gardening. In many places co-ops are available, and these result in considerable savings. Farmers' markets are becoming more prevalent, and not only do shoppers get fresh produce there at lower prices but looking at the stalls is a pleasant open-air experience. Of course, shopping and cooking are always individual matters; but the nurse can encourage clients to use food guides and marketing lists and to take time to prepare a best-for-your-money list of their own.

The following table is an example of a low-cost weekly market order for a couple 55 to 75 years of age.

TABLE 13-1

Kind of Food	Man	Woman
Milk, cheese, ice cream, or milk equivalent	3½ qt	3½ qt
Meat, fish, or poultry	3 lbs	2 lb 8 oz
Eggs	6	5
Dry peas and beans; nuts.	4 oz	4 oz
Grain products—whole grain, enriched, or restored (flour equivalent).	2 lb 12 oz	2 lb
Citrus fruits, tomatoes	1 lb 12 oz	2 lb
Dark green and deep yellow vegetables	12 oz	1 lb
Potatoes	2 lb 4 oz	1 lb 4 oz
Other fruits and vegetables	4 lb 8 oz	3 lb 12 oz
Fats and oils.	10 oz	4 oz
Sugar and sweets.	10 oz	6 oz

(One pound of bread or baked goods equals $\frac{2}{3}$ lb of flour or cereal.)[11]

The nurse's goal can be to help her clients select a diet free from deficiencies, with plenty of room for individual preference, and to take pride and find enjoyment in the process.

Planning ahead and shopping with a list, the nurse can suggest, is in itself a money-saver. Half of all items purchased are "impulse items," and often these take money which should be allocated for essential foods. It is unwise to shop when you are hungry, for you will buy more than you need. Overbuying, indeed, is a habit which many elderly adults find hard to break when someone in the habit of cooking for a good-sized family now shops for two only, or even one. The family recipes need to be revised so they can be prepared in small quantity, or so that part can be frozen for another time, or so that leftovers can be cut down.

Leftovers, of course, can represent a real saving, a real challenge to culinary creativity, and a real opportunity for variety. A few leftover cooked vegetables will add interest to the next day's salad, casserole, or omelet. Leftover baked beans can be mashed, spiced, and spread on bread for a tasty sandwich. Leftover meats and vegetables can be chopped and warmed up in a simple creamed sauce, varied sometimes by the addition of grated cheese; spices, chives, or parsley from your own kitchen-growing plant all add variety. But it is to be remembered that leftovers require refrigeration and even then should not be kept too long, because food value decreases and danger of food contamination increases as time passes.

Finally, the emergency shelf is a helpful suggestion. This will probably not be a new idea; most housekeepers are in the habit of having one, generally to provide for unexpected guests. This is not the main reason, however, for the older adult; it may be inability to get to the store because of bad weather, a sudden illness, or something of that sort. The emergency shelf gives reassurance. What may well be new to older adults is limited space. If a housekeeper has moved from a house with a big kitchen to a small apartment, the nurse can give good advice as to what items are most important for the emergency shelf. If the client has a freezer, meat, bread, vegetables, and fruit are all available; cheese also can be frozen, though it will be crumbly when it is thawed. But without refrigeration there are many possibilities: canned tuna, salmon, chicken, nonfat dry milk solids, evaporated milk, whole grain cereals, peanut butter, dried peas or beans, dried fruit, cans of soup and vegetables, canned fruit and fruit juices, luncheon meats, pork and beans, corned beef hash, and beef stew. On a judicious selection from this list, a client could get along nicely for a week or two without having to go out. But the nurse should point out that at regular intervals the emergency shelf items should be used up and replaced with new ones.

ROLES OF THE NURSE

The role of the nurse is twofold: dietary assessment and dietary counseling. The nurse has in addition to her dietary assessment skills two important areas of information: knowledge of what is a desirable diet for clients in general in this age group and knowledge of the circumstances, physiological and environmental, of each individual client.

Most elderly people have time on their hands—too much time. While many are "set in their ways," some are looking for new ways to fill their days, a new skill to learn and take pride in. Information and interest about diet and nutrition can open up an interesting and important field for the older adult. An elderly couple can be encouraged to spend a leisurely morning in the supermarket, conferring, consulting their lists, comparing prices, noting new products, finally leaving in mild triumph, prepared to competently meet the nutritional needs of the upcoming week. The clients will not only be eating a better and more varied diet, and therefore will be feeling better, but are finding some new interest in life.

It is important that the nurse be knowledgeable about the resources in the community available in this area. Some places today have "Dial-a-Dietitian," where questions on nutrition can be answered. In other areas, dietitians can be reached through local hospitals, extension services, or public health departments. As we all know, the proportion of senior citizens is steadily increasing in our society; and we also all know that we will eventually find ourselves in that group. Society is taking more and more interest in finding ways not merely to care for them grudgingly as used-up pensioners, but to respect them as people and help them keep their own self-respect and independence. Everything the nurse does to help clients better handle the fundamental matter of what they eat contributes to this admirable and essential end.

BIBLIOGRAPHY

1* Deutsch, Ronald M.: *The Family Guide to Better Food and Better Health*, Bantam Books, Inc., New York, 1973.

2 Williams, Sue Rodwell: *"Essentials of Nutritional Status in the Aging and the Aged As a Component of Public Health Programs,"* A Position Paper, American Public Health Association, Washington, D.C., 1972.

3 Watkins, D. M.: "The Assessment of Nutritional Status in the Aging and the Aged As a Component of Public Health Programs," A Position Paper, American Public Health Association, Washington, D.C., 1972.

4 Watson, D. H., and G. V. Mann (Eds.): "Nutrition and Aging Parts I and II," *Amer. J. C. Nutrition*, 25: 805–859, 1972; 26: 1095–1162, 1973.

5 Mayer, Jean: "Aging and Nutrition," *Geriatrics*, May 1974, pp. 57–59.

6   Food and Nutrition Board, *Recommended Daily Dietary Allowances*, Revised 1973, National Academy of Sciences-National Research Council, Washington, D.C., 1973.

7   *Ten State Nutrition Survey*, 1968–1970, *Highlights*, Department of Health, Education & Welfare Publication No. (HSM) 72-8134. U.S. Department of Health, Education and Welfare, Center for Disease Control, Atlanta, Ga., 1972.

8   Krehl, Willard: "The Influence of Nutritional Environment on Aging," *Geriatrics*, May 1974, pp. 69–75.

9   Harris, P. L., et al.: "Blood Tocopherol Values in Normal Human Adults and Incidence of Vitamin E Deficiency," *Proc. Soc. Exper. Biol. Med.* 107: 351–383, 1967.

10   *Lamy, Peter P.:* "Aging: How Human Physiology Responds," in Ewald W. Busse (ed.), Theory and Therapeutics of Aging, Medcone (Medcom Medical Update Series), New York, 1973.

11* *Food Guide for Older Folks*, U.S. Department of Agriculture, Home and Garden Bulletin No. 17, Superintendent of Documents, 1963.

12* "To Your Health . . .In Your Second Fifty Years," National Dairy Council, Chicago, Ill., 60606, 1975.

13* Troll, Lillian E.: "Eating and Aging," in Virginia M. Brantl and Sister Marie Raymond Brown (Eds.), *Reading in Gerontology*, The C. V. Mosby Company, St. Louis, 1973.

*Starred items are of particular interest.

CHAPTER 14

Sexuality and the Older Adult

There is no group more widely discriminated against in terms of their sexuality than the old. Cultural attitudes which have been responsible for the abundance of myths related to other stages in the life cycle spawn an additional set pertaining to the (allegedly) sexless years after 65. Youth is generally disdainful of sexual interest in the elderly. Authors writing about the "third sex" point out that society has attached a neutral gender to all persons who have reached an average age of 60.[1] The myth of the sexless years becomes a self-fulfilling prophecy for some. Others, continuing to experience a strong sex desire, may feel guilt and shame because they believe they are "oversexed." What is labeled virility at age 25 becomes lechery at age 65.[2] Masturbation, which may have been practiced as a means of relieving sexual tension for half a century, suddenly becomes "infantile." And, symptomatic of our times, old people are generally reticent to discuss their sexual problems, while young people who have no knowledge of the problems do all the talking. In short, the "sexual revolution" has come 50 years too late for the majority of older adults, who are locked into beliefs and practices a lifetime in the making.

PHYSIOLOGY AND BEHAVIOR

With the exception of specific existing diseases, physiological changes do not ring a mandatory curtain on sexuality in either sex.[3] While it may be true that some individuals look forward to a respectable reason to terminate their sex lives, it is most likely because of personal preference, and not because of any physiological reality. There appears to be no biological limitation to sexual capacity in the aging female. And changes experienced by the male do not need to contribute substantially to the diminution of his satisfactory sexual expression.

In fact, the older man has certain advantages over the younger one because his ejaculatory control is much greater. The level of tactile response of the penis decreases, and he is slower to achieve an erection, but he can maintain it for a considerably longer time without feeling the ejaculatory urgency that plagues younger men.[4] And while he may lose his erection rapidly after ejaculation, he is capable of prolonged periods of intercourse as long as he contains his level of arousal at the level below ejaculatory inevitablility.

Masters and Johnson emphasize that at no time in a man's life does he lose the capability of erection, except in rare instances involving injury to or pathology of the central nervous system.[5] In one study, 65 percent of men 75 years and older reported continuing involuntary morning erections, although the average per week declined.[6] The man capable of nocturnal or early-morning erections clearly has no physiological barrier to erection. It is true that after about age 50, secondary impotence increases with each decade. But the man can be trained out of it in most instances, assuming he has adequate health, an available partner, and a sexually stimulating climate.

Among men past 50, it is not uncommon as part of the aging process, for the prostate to become enlarged. Yet even if surgery is required, the majority of men who were potent beforehand retain their potency afterwards, although they may have to adjust to retrograde ejaculation. The most important factor in a man's retaining his sexual ability after prostate surgery is a willing sexual partner.[7]

Research coming out of the Duke University Center for the Study of Aging and Human Development reports finding sexually active individuals in every decade under 100 years. In one sample of 254 subjects, approximately 80 percent of aging men (average age, 68 years) continued to be interested in sex and about 70 percent of the same age group were still regularly sexually active. By the time they reached age 78, there was almost no loss of interest, but the proportion of those still regularly sexually active had declined to about 25 percent.[8] Other reported studies attest to the constancy of the sex drive throughout life. Of seventy-four men whose average age was 71, 75 percent still had sexual desire, and 55 percent retained sexual capability ranging from three or more experiences per week to once every 2 months.[9] Of 104 men aged 75 to 92 responding to a questionnaire sent out by *Sexology* magazine, almost half reported that coitus was still satisfactory; six of these men engaged in it more than eight times a month.[10]

The sexual behavior of aging women is less well reported. In the Duke studies, women showed less interest in sex, and a smaller proportion reported continuing activity. In contrast to the men in the sample, marital status made a lot of difference in the sexual expression of women, with very few unmarried women reporting any degree of regular sexual activity in the later years.[11] The unavailability of a socially sanctioned sexual partner was the principal determinant for the discontinuation of sexual activity on the part of many women, which, given the disparity in life expectancy, raises the possibility that their reported decrease in interest in sexual activity may be a defense mechanism to protect them against what they understand to be the inevitable.

In view of the findings about female sexuality coming out of the Duke studies, the ratio of available older men to available older women is highly significant. Pfeiffer provides a concrete demonstration of the imbalance of numbers as he describes one housing project for the elderly.

> The residents were 375 people aged 65 or older—75 men and 300 women, for a ratio of 400:100. 73 of these men were married; only 2 were unmarried. That leaves 2 available men for 227 women. Thus although biology may not limit the sexual capabilities of aging women, it does restrict their opportunities for sexual expression through the limits biology sets on the survival of males.[3]

Another important finding from the Duke studies is that the likelihood of continued sexual expression in the later years is substantially greater for persons who have been highly interested and highly sexually active in their younger years.[11] (Thus, "If you don't use it, you lose it" would seem to be more accurate than the contention that "you can wear it out.") This tendency is important for nurses wishing to respect the continuation of life-style for every aged person. While it would be inappropriate to insist on new or uncongenial patterns of sexual expression in aging clients, it is highly desirable to encourage and assure continuity of sexual expression for those for whom this has consituted an important part of their lives in the past.

THE NEED FOR INTIMACY

A drive for close, intimate contact with another human being is built in at birth and never diminishes in intensity or meaningfulness. Throughout the life cycle, we long for human beings to respond to us — whether by engagement of the mind and emotions as experienced in sharing intellectual exchange, joys, and sorrows, or by engagement of the body as found in touching, patting, stroking, hugging, and sometimes, sexual intercourse. In actuality, many obvious needs such as food and shelter are secondary in importance to that for intimacy and warmth shared with another person who needs and is needed by us. It is little wonder, then, that old people, frequently deprived of their mates through having outlived them, separated from family members both in terms of physical and emotional distance as a result of our mobile population with its emphasis on nuclear families, separated from meaningful employment by mandatory retirement, and experiencing increasing dependence because of chronic health problems and reduced income, should have tremendous needs for some expression of affection and concern from another human being. Their efforts to attain some semblance of physical closeness by touching must be viewed, then, not as unhealthy or obscene, but as an expression of a normal human drive, and a plea for recognition.

Old people can become very ingenious in their efforts to reach out to touch and be touched by the young; observe the delight of older people as they cuddle and stroke infants and toddlers. As long as their overtures aren't blatantly sexual, they are tolerated with some amount of charity, even amusement. But when the touching behavior extends to include older children and other adults, unless it involves immediate family members, it mysteriously becomes unacceptable. As at all other stages in the life cycle, we tend to be generally more comfortable with older women engaging in touching behavior than with older men. While there are some variations depending on cultural orientation, these values tend to be found in the majority of American communities. The stereotype of the old man who molests children persists in spite of the fact that their numbers are negligible when compared to the young male adult molester.[12, 13]

We know from the research data that sexual needs are integral to being human and that for people in their sixties, seventies, and eighties, there is no intrinsic physiological basis for their not being met. These needs may be felt in sexual forms or in "parasexual" ways, such as hunger for simple expressions of affection such as touching, kissing, and embracing. Behavior, however, which in young adults may be acceptable and natural is looked upon with curiosity, suspicion, and disapproval when it appears in older adults. The old man who reaches out to pat the buttocks of his young female attendant is often labeled an "old fool making a pass." Had he been 50 years younger, he would have still been making a pass, but he would no longer be a fool.[13] The behavior of the women residents who flirt over a game of cards with the one available ambulatory male in the nursing home is described by the amused staff as ridiculous and out of place for anyone "their age." Most people could acknowledge that they are aware of the continuing existence of the "oldest profession in the world," yet would be shocked to hear a group of men at a conference on aging discussing the practice of prostitution by elderly women in a retirement community, and even further horrified to hear the men joking about recommending that particular community over others because that service was available.

As health care professionals, we should concern ourselves with providing the security, support, and privacy needed to nurture and conserve relationships in which older clients are likely to be able to satisfy the basic human drive for intimacy. In reality, as well as discounting the possibility of continuing sexual feelings in old people, we tend to discourage their expression by using the guise of institutional rules and regulations, treatment priorities, schedules, fear of exploitation of the "victim," and concern about propriety and public opinion.

VIGNETTE

The staff of the nursing home was in an uproar. The new resident, 83-year-old Matthew, was outrageously flirtatious, and had been observed pinching Millie, age 79, and Tina, age 84, on the buttocks. The dayroom had been buzzing with an unaccustomed excitement for the past week. None of the patients had complained, but the staff felt that Matthew's behavior would have to be curtailed or he would cause all the old ladies to be upset.

One might legitimately ask who had the problem? Staff, and very often family members, become uncommonly upset when their expectations of a sexual behavior in older clients are not met. It is highly likely that each of us has much difficulty dealing with the possibility that our own parents, let alone our grandparents, are sexual beings, and that we generalize that conflict to all older adults. Burnside stresses that professionals can be more instrumental in promoting a healthful attitude and milieu for the aged if they have their own attitudes and feelings in control.[2] Nurses should consider how they might manipulate the environment to allow clients more opportunity to express their sexuality. Institutional based professionals could learn something from senior citizen centers. Socialization among the sexes can be encouraged by participation in card parties, afternoon coffee, beer or sherry hours, or cooking meals together. Dancing is another social activity that can provide close contact.

Nurses should also consider whether or not they could be more courageous about intervention on behalf of the elderly in matters of their sexuality. Segregation of the sexes and the absence of double beds in most nursing homes in effect may defy 40 to 50 years of sleeping habits for old couples who are admitted together. Nurses can assume the position of client advocate, encouraging that rigid rules be bent to accommodate to individual needs. Nurses could accept responsibility for modifying the environment by something as uncomplicated as wiring two single beds together. It is quite inhumane and totally nonproductive to simply chart "Patient confused and disoriented" when some ingenious client, in search of his mate, satisfies his own need for closeness by climbing into an already occupied bed. And given that we are extremely uncomfortable with heterosexual activity in the aged, it is probably safe to say that the needs of the aged client with a homosexual preference are totally ignored. It is beyond the scope of this chapter to deal with potential remedies for that "Pandora's box."

ALTERNATIVES TO INTERCOURSE

As at every other developmental stage of the life cycle, there are alternatives available (albeit seldom discussed) when intercourse is no longer possible. Since women commonly outlive their men, they tend to face longer periods when a socially sanctioned sex partner is no longer available. People who continue to have a sex drive but not act on it may deal with the need by sublimation, or engaging in other activities in an effort to decrease the tension without directly satisfying the need.

Fantasy may be an acceptable outlet for dealing with sexual need. Considerable interest has been recently generated in the content of women's sexual fantasies, and some therapists are even using the fantasy experience as a tool to reverse sexual dysfunction or enhance sexual experience for people of all ages. The nurse may need to keep in mind that fantasizing, while considered a perfectly normal form of entertainment, may not be totally acceptable to the older person unless specific permission is given.

Masturbation continues to be a viable form of sexual expression for the old. But given the existing societal expectations of a lack of interest in sex among the old, masturbation is no better tolerated than heterosexual behavior among this age group, particularly if it occurs at an "inappropriate" time or place.

VIGNETTE

78-year old Max needed assistance into the tub from his young attendant, but was able to bathe himself. One morning she discovered him masturbating in the tub. She became flustered and ordered him to "cut that out," then fled the scene.

The attendant's opinion was that masturbation is okay—in bed, under the covers, alone, at night, with the lights out. In discussing this incident with her supervising nurse, the attendant was able to recognize that she might have responded to Max's behavior more therapeutically. One way would be to acknowledge that Max needed some privacy right now and suggest that he put his light on when he was ready to be assisted out of the tub. This would convey her acceptance of the legitimacy of his behavior, yet let him know that her expectation was that it should take place in privacy.

It is important to reassert that each client has a right to personal preference. Rubin points out that for those who are ready and willing to give up sexual relations, perhaps the wisest course is graceful acceptance of the ending of sexual activity.[14] In effect, they choose to lay their sex lives to psychic rest. These clients have a right to be supported in their decision and to be free from persuasive arguments advanced by "liberal" health care professionals.

CHRONIC DISEASE AND SEXUAL EXPRESSION

A number of illnesses, physical or mental, can temporarily lead to a decrease or even disappearance of sexual expression. The restriction of sexual activity as a result of physical infirmities is frequently increased by iatrogenic factors such as health care professionals failing to give necessary guidance or overtly giving negative or discouraging advice. Nurses must be careful not to feed into the client's anxiety in these ways. For example, a depressive reaction may interrupt the desire for sex, but once successfully treated, the client should not expect any permanent effect on his pre-illness level of libido. Similarly, once a myocardial infarction has healed, there is no reason why the cardiac patient should not return to his regular sexual expression, unless he is so severely impaired that he cannot tolerate even modest exercise.[3] Anemia, glandular dysfunction, or malnutrition may cause excessive fatigue and result in decreased libido. If the cause is correctly diagnosed and treated, the client's sexual problems should be easily reversed.

The cardiac patient and his partner should understand that sexual activity always increases the heart rate, blood pressure, and breathing rate at the point of orgasm and ejaculation and then these subside rapidly. Research indicates the average maximal heart rate for older men is around 120 beats and lasts 10 to 15 seconds.[15] However, other activities of daily living, such as driving a car, arguments, physical and mental work, and any frustrating situation or conflicting emotions may require as much or more of the heart as does sex. One rule of thumb is that if the client can climb two flights of stairs without experiencing prolonged breathlessness and heart palpitations, he should be able to tolerate intercourse.[16]

Sexual activity for the client with heart disease should be avoided in situations of fatigue resulting from mental and physical activity; after heavy eating or drinking; in an uncomfortable temperature; and after an argument, especially an unresolved one. There are several ways to make sexual activity less demanding on the heart: Take a half-hour nap before and after; have sex in the morning, shortly after waking, to avoid fatigue; avoid bearing the partner's weight by lying supine with the partner kneeling above; sit facing the partner on an armless chair, low enough to allow the feet to firmly touch the floor; or use a face-to-face side lying position.[17]

Chronic degenerative diseases such as diabetes can have an effect on sexual capacity and interest. The elderly male diabetic commonly experiences progressive erectile impotence and the female may become inorgasmic due to peripheral neuropathy. These dysfunctions are irreversible. Although there has been some work done on methods of surgical splinting for the male, the techniques have not been perfected.

Aches and pains in the lower back and limbs may be attributed to coitus when in reality they result from postural defects or musculoskeletal pathology (e.g., osteoporosis). Muscle relaxants and analgesics can be prescribed for comfort and vitamin B complex will relieve much of the neuritis which triggers the muscle spasms.[18]

Patients with arthritis should be advised to premeditate and premedicate, and may take the following measures: They should plan to have sex during the part of the day when they feel most rested, relaxed, and free of pain. Techniques for relaxation such as hot packs, hot showers, a drink, or listening to music should be used in preparing for sex. Principles of joint protection should apply when choosing a position—rear entry is found to be very comfortable by many arthritic women. A lubricant such as K-Y jelly facilitates easy entry of the penis into the vagina, and analgesics taken about 20 minutes before coitus begins reduce discomfort. Finally, a vibrator may be useful for the arthritic person who enjoys touching but is no longer able to massage the partner.[19]

URINARY TRACT PROBLEMS IN WOMEN

The incidence of urinary tract infections in women is directly related to sexual activity. Older sexually active women are particularly susceptible to urologic problems because of physical changes related to aging. Weakened urethral and vaginal walls, diminished vaginal lubrication, and a more constricted, shorter vaginal barrel predispose postmenopausal women to trauma and mechanical irritation during intercourse. Therefore, urinary infections such as cystitis, urethritis, and cystourethritis are more likely to occur when sexual intercourse takes place, although, given the tendency for sexual intercourse to decrease in frequency as women grow older, the overall incidence of such disorders is likely to decrease.

Another factor probably associated with the origin of urologic problems in older women is the tendency of their partners, because of delayed ejaculatory response, to engage in extended periods of intercourse. This practice brings mixed blessings to the woman, for, while it may increase her pleasure, it increases the likelihood that infecting bacteria may be "massaged" into the paraurethral glands, from which they can move to the bladder to cause cystitis.

As a rule, infections originating during sexual intercourse are manifested about 36 hours later. Their treatment differs from non-infectious urologic disorders, thus requiring a urine culture and perhaps one or two other tests to obtain a differential diagnosis. The purpose of this therapy is, obviously, to eradicate bacteria from the urinary tract. Nurses should be alert to the fact that it is fairly common for urethritis and cystitis to recur regularly despite extensive antibacterial treatment. Clients with this health problem need to be instructed in various techniques to help prevent recurrent infections. Since it is assumed that bacteria are pushed into the urologic tract by sexual intercourse, it may be helpful for the patient to flush out the lower urinary tract by urinating as soon as possible after intercourse. Intake of extra fluids may facilitate this. A shower or bath prior to intercourse may decrease the number of organisms in the periurethral area. The male-superior position for intercourse is probably not advisable when recurrent infection is a problem, because this position exerts extra stress on the urethra.[20]

Another fairly common disorder in postmenopausal women is genital relaxation. Instead of a dry, inelastic canal, the large relaxed vagina is often overlubricated by seeping cervical erosions. A cystocele, bladder incontinence, rectocele, or uterine prolapse causes obvious difficulties during intercourse.[18] While surgical correction may be indicated, one conservative measure is for the client to practice the Kegel exercises. These are a series of repetitive exercises to develop the pubococcygenus muscle; these exercises involve systematic tightening and relaxing the muscles as if stopping and starting urination.[21]

Although the discomfort of urinary disorders certainly interferes with optimal enjoyment of sex, it is rarely serious enough to require sexual abstinence, except as a temporary form of therapy. Nurses should be aware that the woman who uses urologic problems as a convenient excuse to forego sex entirely requires exploration of the inadequacy of her sexual experience as well as the medical aspects of her urologic disorder.

SEXUAL DYSFUNCTION IN OLD AGE

Therapy for the sexual and marital problems of the elderly should include a thorough medical exam, treatment for any physical abnormalities and their psychosomatic complaints, and counseling for both partners concerning the psychological aspects of the problem.[18]

Many clients seek special vitamins or other substances which can improve their potency. No special diet is of any use in restoring potency, and the so-called "aphrodesiac" foods operate by the power of suggestion only. Some drugs have the effect of heightening sexual experience (e.g., amyl nitrite inhaled at the point of orgasm, strychnine, L-dopa) but they are dangerous unless prescribed and directed by a physician. Herbs and spices may be used to irritate the lining of the genitourinary tract, causing a vague genital urge and reflex erection, but they usually don't increase sexual drive. The most effective aphrodesiacs are good health, plenty of rest and sleep, adequate exercise, and freedom from emotional tension.[22]

There is a thriving mail-order business in mechanical devices, such as plaster molds, splints, suction devices, and clasps, designed to treat impotence. The use of artificial devices should not be summarily dismissed by health care professionals; little is known or documented about their efficacy. While they may be expensive, if they help a man to improve his sexual function, they may be well worth the price. Some counselors suggest that an ordinary rubber band placed around the base of the penis after erection has been attained is equally effective and clearly much less expensive. However, this measure does require that a man achieve at least a partial erection.

Nurses counseling elderly couples should try to work towards attitudinal changes and improving the nature of the interpersonal relationship — not just teach the couple about available "gimmicks." It is important for nurses to encourage communication focused on the "here and now" and avoid the rehashing of old painful experiences. The prognosis is poor for couples who have developed a pattern of dysfunctional communication over the years and then are faced with sexual problems.

CONCLUSION

It has been said that successfully aging persons are those who have made a decision to stay in training in major areas of their lives, including that of sexuality.[3] To help improve the quality of life in later years, it is important, therefore, that older people be helped to attain the creative expression of their sexuality for the purpose of "satisfying their particular emotional needs in accordance with their current physical abilities and interpersonal relationships."[14]

We have seen that the expression of sexuality includes, but is not limited to, sexual intercourse. It also manifests itself in a tone of voice, a sense of humor, a touch, or a demonstration of overt affection, such as a hug. We have also seen that chronological age is no barrier to the continued sexual life of the old when opportunity and saction are present.

It seems highly appropriate to conclude this chapter with Jacobson's bill of rights for guaranteeing sexual freedom.[23]

- *The right to express yourself as a sexual being.*
- *The right to be self-confident and self-directing in regard to your sexuality.*
- *The right to become the person you would like to be.*
- *The right to select and be with a sex partner of your choice, whether it be of the same sex or of the opposite sex.*
- *The right to be aware of the influence your sexuality can have on someone else and to use it in a constructive and therapeutic manner.*
- *The right to encourage your peer group members to function as sexual beings.*
- *The right to assist others in asserting and expressing their sexuality.*
- *The right to be accepting and tolerant of another's sexual attitudes and preferences.*
- *The right to assist men and women of all ages to recognize their sexuality as an integral part of their personality, inherited at conception, molded and tempered by environment, sustained by health, threatened by disease, and reversed by choice.*

Thus, we reaffirm our position that sexuality is a quality of personality, and that the sex drive is a normal phenomenon experienced throughout the life cycle, up to and including old age.

BIBLIOGRAPHY

1. Masters, W. H., and J. W. Ballew: "The Third Sex," *Geriatrics*, 10:1-4, 1955.
2. Burnside, Irene Mortenson: "Sexuality and Aging," *Med. Arts & Sciences*, 27(3):13-27, 1973.
3. Pfeiffer, Eric: "Sexuality in the Aging Individual," *J. Amer. Geriat. Soc.*, 22(11):481-484, 1974.
4. McCary, James Leslie: *Human Sexuality*, Van Nostrand Reinhold Company, New York, 1973.
5. Masters, W. H., and Virginia Johnson: *Human Sexual Inadequacy*, Little, Brown and Company, Boston, 1970.
6. Rubin, Isadore: "Sex Over Sixty-Five," H. G. Beigel (ed.), in *Advance in Sex Research*, pp. 138-142, Harper & Row, Publishers, Incorporated, New York, 1963.
7. Finkle, A. L.: "Sex After Prostatectomy," *Med. Aspects Human Sexuality*, II(3):40-41, 1968.
8. Pfeiffer, Eric, A. Verwoerdt, and H. S. Wang: "Sexual Behavior in Aged Men and Women. I. Observations of 254 Community Volunteers," *Arch. Gen. Psychiat.* 19:753-758, 1968.
9. Freeman, J. T.: "Sexual Capacities in the Aging Male," *Geriatrics* 16:37-43, 1961.
10. Tarail, M.: "Sex Over 65," *Sexology*, 28:440-445, 1962.
11. Pfeiffer, Eric, and Glenn C. Davis: "Determinants of Sexual Behavior in Middle and Old Age," *J. Amer. Geriat. Soc.*, 20(4):151-158, 1972.
12. Epstein, L. J., C. Mills, and A. Simon: "Antisocial Behavior in the Elderly," *Comp. Psychiat.*, 2(1):36-42, 1970.
13. Weinberg, Jack: "Sexual Expression in Late Life," *Amer. J. Psychiat.* 126(5):713-716, 1969.
14. Rubin, Isadore: "Sex and Aging, Man and Woman," in Clark E. Vincent (ed.), *Human Sexuality in Medical Education and Practice*, pp. 517-531, Charles C. Thomas, Publishers, Springfield, Ill., 1968.
15. Hellerstein, H. K., and E. H. Friedman: "Sexual Activity and the Post Coronary Patient," *Arch. Intern. Med.*, 125:987-999, 1970.
16. Wagner, Nathaniel: "Sexual Activity and the Cardiac Patient," in *Human Sexuality: a Health Practitioner's Text*, Richard Green (ed.), The Williams & Wilkins Company, Baltimore, 1975.
17. Griffith, George: "Sexuality and the Cardiac Patient," *Heart Lung: J. Critical Care*, 2:70-73, 1973.
18. Kavinoky, Nadina: "Counseling the Marital and Sexual Problems of Older Patients," in Richard H. Klemer (ed.), *Counseling the Marital and Sexual Problems: A Physician's Handbook*, pp. 167-176, Williams & Wilkins Company, Baltimore, 1965.
19. Lachniet, Donna, and Jan Onder: *Sex and Arthritis and Women*, paper presented at the 8th Scientific Session, Allied Health Professions Section, the Arthritis Foundation, Los Angeles, June 1973.
20. Kent, Saul: "Urinary Tract Problems in Women Are Linked to Sexual Activity," *Geriatrics*, 30(7):145-146, 1975.
21. Kegel, A. H.: "Sexual Functions of the Pubococcygeus Muscle," *West. J. Surg.*, 60:521-524, 1952.

22. Rubin, Isadore: "Sex after 40 — and After 70," in R. Brecher and E. Brecher (eds.), *An Analysis of Human Sexual Response*, New American Library, Inc., New York, 1966.

23. Jacobson, Linbania: "Illness and Human Sexuality," *Nursing Outlook*, 22(1) 50–53, 1974.

24. Christenson, Cornelia, and John Gagnon: "Sexual Behavior in a Group of Older Women," *J. Gerontol.*, 203:351–356, 1965.

25. Pease, Ruth A.: "Female Professional Students and Sexuality in the Aging Male," *Gerontologist*, 14(2):153–157, 1974.

26. Rubin, Isadore: *Sexual Life After Sixty*, Basic Books, Inc., Publishers, New York, 1965.

27. Rubin, Isadore: *Sexual Life in the Later Years*. SIECUS Study Guide No. 12, 1970.

28. Dickinson, Peter: *The Fires of Autumn: Sexual Activity in the Middle and Later Years*. Drake Publishers, Inc., New York, 1974.

CHAPTER 15

Managing Retirement

Retirement can be viewed as an event, a process, or a social adjustment. Many gerontologists feel it is the most crucial life change for the older adult.[1] Perhaps the nurse may be of most help to clients in this field by helping them to look at it as a second career: by suggesting they prepare for it ahead of time and put thought, care, and effort into making a success of it. By this time of life, clients have learned that this is the price of making a success of any worthwhile undertaking.

RETIREMENT PROCESS

Retirement, obviously, means a change in the way of life. Both the retiree and spouse (if a spouse exists) need to develop attitudes, values, and skills suitable to the new way. As is true of almost anything, finances have a strong influence upon this period and the decisions necessitated by it. *Before anything else*, clients must know where they will stand in regard to retirement income.

One decision a person must make about retirement is *when*. This may or may not be the choice of the person involved. As of now, only one person in ten is forced to retire by reaching a mandatory age; but this proportion is increasing and will probably increase even more in the future, particularly since present retirement ages will almost certainly be lowered. Mandatory retirement is universal in government employment, and many firms have this policy. The age can range from 55 to 70, but retirement before 65 generally means reduced postretirement benefits.

That a mandatory policy exists probably influences voluntary retirement before the age limit. Research in the 1950s found poor health was the most prevalent reason. But a more recent study (1965) found it the reason in only a quarter of the cases. Nearly 70 percent of early retirees felt they could afford to quit, or wanted more free time.[2] The desire for leisure is becoming a more and more popular reason.

There is no evidence to indicate that retirement hastens death. "He was just fine till he retired; then he had nothing to do, and a year later he was dead"; this is a common notion, but a fallacy. Poor health may be a cause for retirement, but our evidence indicates that retired persons are in as good health after retirement as before, or sometimes better.[3]

It is impossible to name an ideal age for retirement since it is largely an individual matter, and since finances play a large part. Some people must work as long as they can; others need not. Some enjoy their work so much they never want to leave it; others can hardly wait for the last day. It seems safe to say, however, that tapering off is preferable to a sudden break. Perhaps, if it is possible, it is a good idea to gradually increase the length of the annual vacation or reduce the length of the working day. At present most people who retire suddenly do so because of unexpected illness or an unexpected economic emergency, such as failure of the firm where they are employed, reduction in personnel, or the like. Some people not regularly employed may find it hard to get jobs as they grow older, and may therefore retire. Employers sometimes discriminate against the elderly, alleging they cannot meet job requirements, though often there is no foundation for these allegations.

A second retirement decision is *living arrangements*, which may or may not involve change.

VIGNETTE

Tony and Barbara have lived for 23 years in their own home, which they own free and clear, in a desirable neighborhood of a middle-class suburb of a large city. Taxes have risen because of this desirability, and because of inflation. When Tony retires, which will be soon, they are doubtful whether or not they can afford to keep on living in their own house.

It is a comfort to live in your own home and near old neighbors, who can be trusted to come in and help in case of illness or emergency. If Tony and Barbara have to move, can they find a place where they will be so happy? Can they make new friends at their age? On the other hand, as they grow older, their house (in which they brought up three children, now grown) may seem too large: too many stairs to climb, too many rooms to clean. Would an apartment be better? Would a milder climate be more pleasant? In their Northern state, winters are long and cold. In a Southern one, heating bills would be low, there would be no snow to shovel, and they could spend more time outdoors and have a long gardening season. For a Northerner, moving to the South can reduce living expenses considerably, since housing, taxes, and payment for services (house painting, dry cleaning, household help) are usually lower there. The same thing would hold true in moving from a city suburb to a small town.

Perhaps some of Tony and Barbara's old neighbors have died or moved away and the houses have been taken by families with motorcycle-riding teenagers. Perhaps they could move where there would be more people of their own age, with congenial tastes. In a new neighborhood they might feel free to try a few new ways of living frowned on in their old community. They have always enjoyed the cultural resources of a big city; might it be pleasant to go to a small town where entertainment takes the form of church suppers and informal get-togethers? (At the same time that Tony and Barbara are pondering these questions, there may be another couple of the same age who have always lived in a small town and are wondering whether they might not enjoy moving to a city where they can visit art galleries, museums, plays, and concerts, and have some of the cultural experiences not now available to them.) And finally, if they decide to move, how far away from their old home should they go? If the distance is too great, it is unlikely that old friends—and even their children—will have the time or money to visit them often.

No one, certainly not the nurse, can make the decision for them; but the nurse can encourage them to consider the whole matter very carefully, with all its pros and cons. And the nurse is in a position to give indispensable health advice. Some clients would feel much better in a warm, dry climate; others must avoid high altitudes. One of the very most important considerations in reaching this decision, surely, is in what surroundings they will feel, physically, at their best.

Where to Live When You Retire, by Margery Mack, is a helpful booklet the nurse can recommend.[4]   She gives the following advice:

1 Don't sell your home until you are sure where you want to settle.
2 Investigate the advantages and disadvantages of several locations before you decide on the best for you.
3 Rent for a year before you buy or build in the community of your choice.
4 Don't buy impulsively, but count the pros and cons.
5 Be sure the future neighbors are "your kind."
6 Try to make friendships in the new community before you buy or build.

This wise advice underlines the importance of taking nothing for granted without early and thorough investigation. The nurse will have plenty of opportunity to emphasize this. The same principle applies when the topic under discussion is not a move to a new community but to a retirement facility. Does it provide life-long medical care, nursing when necessary, or personal care to the end of life? What does it cost? What type of contract is involved? What are its advantages and disadvantages? All these topics should be thoroughly investigated and individually assessed.

A third decision is *supplementing retirement income*, income which for most people is less than what they have been used to. If it is decided that this is desirable, the next question is *how*.

There are possibilities in part-time employment, postretirement reemployment, or starting a new career. One word of warning: clients should inform themselves of how earning additional income will affect their social security benefits. The nurse should make sure they visit the district social security office and are aware of the latest regulations.

Early preparation for retirement work, like early preparation for retirement living arrangements, pays dividends. Here is an opportunity for some new experiences and mild adventures: a chance to try something one "always wanted to do but never had time for." All sorts of materials are available on how to prepare for job interviews or set up a new business. Preretirement life has developed a considerable capital, so to speak, in abilities, skills, and interests; this is the time to invest this capital in a new and stimulating job or business.[5]

Some possibilities are serving as receptionists, doing accounting, and taking telephone calls for doctors, lawyers, or real estate agencies. There are many possibilities for self-employment: doing sewing and alterations; staging parties and puppet shows for children; putting up box lunches for offices and factories; soliciting by telephone for some product; door-to-door selling; serving as a companion;

furnishing reading and/or shopping service for shut-ins; ghostwriting; typing manuscripts; making jewelry or other crafts; catering; teaching music. The nurse can point out that the amount of money gained should be second in importance; first and foremost, the occupation should be *enjoyed.*

Hobbies sometimes have money-making possibilities: for example, making doll houses or miniature furniture; painting; photography; stamp or coin collecting; dabbling in antiques; growing flowers, herbs, or houseplants; breeding pets, raising canaries and parakeets, raising rabbits; teaching chess or contract; and genealogy and local history research.

Possible positions for older workers are almost endless: automobile mechanic, cook, decorator, filer, locksmith, luggage repairer, piano tuner, cashier, counter clerk, butler, guide, hostess, restaurant worker, caretaker, farm couple, grounds keeper, kennel worker, housekeeper, chauffeur, golf course ranger, delivery person, mother's helper, or house-, pet-, and baby-sitter.

Some such occupation, often part-time, has a great advantage in addition to supplementing income. Up to retirement, workers feel the satisfaction of doing something useful, of contributing to society, and being respected for it. At retirement, they lose this satisfaction, as well as the stimulation of contact with fellow workers from whom they get new ideas and with whom they keep up with new trends. Many retirees, like wound-up alarm clocks, still are set in the habits formed by years of work.[6] Though now they can sleep as late as they want, they wake up at the usual time. Then how to fill the empty hours formerly spent at the office or wherever? Where to go? Whom to talk to? The postretirement job is a good answer.

Apart from gainful employment, there are many activities to fill the void. We have already discussed the role that volunteer work can play in the middle adult's life, and those already involved can merely continue. New activities in which to participate include Foster Grandparents, retired senior volunteer programs, and the American Association of Retired Persons, to mention only a few.[7] Hobbies for the elderly could fill 36 hours a day, from doing the daily crossword in the paper in the morning to the Late Late Show at night; crafts; collecting stamps, coins, portraits, postmarks; weaving; woodworking, painting, lapidary work, photography; games of all sorts, from pinochle and cards to shuffleboard and ringtoss; studying the family tree or becoming an expert on a particular historical period; sports; and hunting, fishing, and sailing. (See Chapter 13 for additional ideas.)

Perhaps the retirement activity par excellence is travel. For countless elders, retirement brings the realization of a life-long ambition: to see Stratford-on-Avon, Kenya, or Paris. They read about their destination beforehand, take the trip (perhaps on a guided tour), and re-live the experience again and again, looking at the pictures and mementos they gather. It is true that travel is among the more expensive recreations, which limits its appeal. But retirees are free to travel out-of-season, when rates are lower, which is an advantage. Many enjoy trailer travel, with its informality and ease. On the other hand, many enjoy staying at home far more than ever before, since they now have plenty of time to devote to the garden and house. Many a man finds his own fresh vegetables the best he has ever eaten; many a woman has special pleasure and pride in redecorating a room herself.

Finally, the process of retirement should include provision for health care. Elderly adults should know to what benefits they are entitled through their particular retirement arrangements or through Medicare. Dental care is rarely covered by health insurance, and the need for dental work is common in this period; the nurse should encourage clients to have it carried out before retirement brings curtailment of income. Catastrophic illness can literally ruin people unprepared for it. In this area, the nurse can help clients assess their medical coverage. She also can inform clients of community services for which they are eligible; these may range from a free walk-in community storefront center to home health care.

In summary, adjustment to retirement is facilitated if people retire voluntarily, taper off work instead of making a clean break, explore postretirement possibilities of all sorts thoroughly, and come to informed decisions. They should plan and prepare ahead of time for the new life as they planned and prepared for their former careers, and work at making it a success.[8]

ROLE CHANGES

Retirement means change. The worker loses not only the work role but also the work-related roles sometimes provided through a union or a professional association. There are new expectations: that more time be spent with family and friends, in leisure, and in organizations not related to work; and that less income be spent. Research indicates that most retired people conform to these expectations.[3]

There is also a significant change in the roles of husband and wife. Spouses spend more time together than previously, and are in general successful or not, in proportion to their development of common interests in the middle years after the children have left home. Other changes occur in the roles of parents. Parents' satisfaction with their children, according to a study done on various aspects of marriage over the life cycle, is highest in the postparental period and then begins to decline. For men, it is lowest during their children's high school years; for women, the grade school years. And the drop during the retirement period is more pronounced for men than for women. If parents have been successful in adapting to their children's growth to adulthood and independence, the relationship will probably continue to be good and satisfying; if they have not, they may face a lonely old age. Women generally have a closer relationship with children than men, but therefore may develop more friction because of the very closeness. If the parent-child relationship is satisfactory up to the age of 50 or 55 for the parent, it is unlikely that new alienation will then develop.[9]

Some elderly persons, however, do depend on their children for companionship, and continue to think of them as children and want to exert parental authority. Grown children resent this. Elderly parents who are happy and have interests of their own are emotionally less dependent on their children, and the nurse encourages elderly clients to develop a variety of new interests.

Grandparenting can also involve role changes. When men and women reach old age, their grandchildren are teenagers or young adults. An unhappy phenomenon is the development of a generation gap—not that between parents and children, which has existed in practically every period of history, but between grandparents and grandchildren. When generations live closely together, friction is even more likely to develop. With our typical American mobility, however, generations often live far apart. Even though many grandparents may see grandchildren comparatively rarely, they can still keep in touch by frequent letters and phone calls and have happy relationships.

The loss of a spouse from divorce or death, but generally from the latter, is a common change in this period. Since men tend to die earlier than women, widowhood is more common than widowerhood. It has been estimated that half of American women over 60 are widows; by the age of 85 the percentage has risen to 85 percent.[8]

Since all adjustments are more difficult to make with increasing age, such a serious loss as the death of a spouse is difficult indeed. Old age sometimes is accompanied by decreasing social interests. Many elderly people assuage their loneliness and receive great comfort from a pet. Remarriages are not infrequent (see Chapter 13).

Studies have shown, however, that satisfaction with the present stage in the family life cycles rises during old age. Thus most older persons, now their parental responsibilities are over and they can enjoy freedom, feel satisfaction with their marriage and their lives, as long as they can be together. We do not have evidence for the idea that marital disenchantment progresses over the life cycle.

Nor do we have evidence for the popular belief that the old person who has never married will face an unhappy and lonely old age. In the course of life, such persons have learned to develop interests and take part in activities which compensate for the lack of a spouse; and in old age, after retirement, these are merely continued.

PRERETIREMENT COUNSELING

The nurse can be of great importance in providing preretirement counseling to older adults. Many programs are already in effect for retiring employees in hospitals, businesses, and unions, varying from a single session on retirement benefits to comprehensive and extensive programs covering all aspects.[10] But employees are sometimes reluctant to attend these because they fear that by doing so they will be pushed into early retirement. The nurse should ask clients what experience of this sort they have had, and make sure they are aware of all the topics they should consider: health-related issues of medical and dental care, exercise, nutrition, mental health, and sexuality; living options, retirement communities, and low income housing; and pension and social security benefits can all be discussed. Written materials concerning preretirement counseling can be obtained from many sources.[11] The nurse should also point out the legal matters to which clients should address themselves: wills, inheritance laws, tax rebates, insurance laws, and consumer rights. These preretirement counseling sessions may be a good time for the nurse to give an idea of the wide range of part-time employment and volunteer opportunities which may be available as well as the resources of the community. Nothing will contribute so much to mental health, and overall health, for the elderly as two simple words: "Keep busy."

Barrett has described what makes an elderly person happy.

> The older person who is financially secure, able to use his free time constructively, happy in his social contacts and able to contribute services to others will find the later longevous period of life truly rewarding. He will retain a superior self-concept, remain highly motivated, rarely become neurotic or psychotic and live out his life happily. He will not suffer from psychosocial deprivation, nor will he become senescent. When one is adequately prepared for retirement, these may truly be the "golden years".[11]

BIBLIOGRAPHY

1 Miller, Stephen J.: "The Social Dilemma of the Aging Leisure Participant," in *Older People and Their Social World*, Arnold M. Rose and Warren A. Peterson (eds.), F. A. Davis, Philadelphia, 1965.

2 Pollman, William A.: "Early Retirement: A Comparison of Poor Health and Other Retirement Factors," *J. Gerontol.*, 26: 41-45, 1971.

3 Atchley, Robert C.: *The Social Forces in Later Life*, Wadsworth Publishing Company, Inc., Belmont, Calif., 1972.

4 Mack, Margery J.: *Where to Live When You Retire*, Industrial Relations Center, The University of Chicago, Chicago, 1966.

5 Ingraham, Mark H.: *My Purpose Holds: Reactions and Experiences in Retirement of TIAA-CREF Annuitants*, Educational Research Division, Teachers Insurance and Annuity Association, College Retirement Equities Fund, New York, 1974.

6 Atchley, Robert C.: "Adjustment to Loss of Job at Retirement," *Int. J. Aging Human Dev.*, 6 (1): 7-15, 1975.

7 Saloshin, H. E.: "Retirement: Promise or Threat?" *Minn. Med.* 57: 632-636, 1974.

8 Hurlock, Elizabeth B.: *Developmental Psychology*, 4th ed., McGraw-Hill Book Company, New York, 1975.

9 Burr, W. R.: "Satisfaction With Various Aspects of Marriage Over the Life Cycle: A Random Middle-Class Sample," *J. Marriage Family*, 32: 29-37, 1970.

10 Conklin, William E.: "Preretirement Counseling," *Hospitals*, 47: 86-88, 1973.

11 Barrett, J. H.: *Gerontological Psychology*, Charles C. Thomas, Publisher, Springfield, Ill.

12 Burnside, Irene: *Psycho-social Nursing Care of the Aged*, McGraw-Hill Book Company, New York, 1973.

*Starred items are of particular interest

Assessment Tool for Preventive Health Care

CHAPTER 16

Preventive Health Care

Many adults do not receive routine preventive health care for a variety of reasons. Young adults feel "too healthy" to need it or they think they can't afford it. What young adults don't realize is that the whole point to preventive care is to maintain their health, which may be threatened by many risk factors. While middle adults are often better able to afford routine physical examinations than younger or older adults, they frequently do not initiate regular, annual exams, because they fear an adverse diagnosis or feel that a complete exam is too expensive when not covered by insurance. Older adults often do not have routine preventive health care because they feel that illness is a consequence of aging and cannot be prevented.

Preventive care involves an annual complete health assessment. This is indispensable and serves several purposes. Properly done, it provides the information which the nurse and doctor must have to establish a health maintenance plan and to prevent crises in the succeeding years. It can identify risk factors: for instance, a young adult who smokes and whose father died of heart disease has a double risk of incurring the disease himself.

The consequences of forgoing routine checkups can be undetected or untreated diseases like hypertension and glaucoma, and these

213

create further health risks for diseases like heart attack, strokes, and blindness. Thus failure to have regular, routine checkups to detect the presence of disease, either undetected or untreated diseases like hypertension, is a risk factor.

Other risk factors which may predispose individuals to certain diseases are hereditary, sex, race, and age. For example, individuals whose blood relatives have had heart disease, diabetes, or cancer have an increased likelihood of inheriting a tendency toward those diseases. Women who have not yet experienced menopause are less likely to have heart attacks than men of the same age due to the presence of estrogen and progesterone in the system. Black Americans have twice the chance of developing hypertension than whites. And finally, 60-year-olds have a greater chance of succumbing to chronic illness than 50-year-olds.

This does not mean it is inevitable that adults will develop a disease because of these factors. In fact, susceptibility to some diseases can actually be decreased if an attempt is made to reduce risk factors and to seek routine, preventive health care. Every adult should have a complete, annual medical exam, and some individuals should have them more often depending on their health history and their physician's recommendations.

A typical physical examination for an adult should include a health history and a physical examination with laboratory studies. Examination of the thyroid gland, mouth, throat, and skin; of the prostate gland in men; the breast and pelvis, including a Pap smear in women, should be included. Vital signs, blood pressure, urinalysis and electrocardiogram for males over 30 and one for both males and females as a baseline, serum cholesterol and triglycerides, and blood tests (CBC., Hct., Sed. Rate, SMA-12, glucose tolerance) should be a part of the health assessment. Middle adults should have a proctoscopy or sigmoidoscopy of the rectum for detection of cancerous polyps. Some physicians recommend a limited chest x-ray, particularly for smokers. The examination should include a review of current immunization status. That includes receiving an up-to-date diptheria and tetanus immunization and a TB skin test when appropriate. Young adult females should have a rubella titer, males a mumps titer, to determine if they have had these diseases. Blacks should be tested for sickle-cell anemia.

The annual physical should be supplemented by vision, dental, and hearing examinations. This is particularly important since periodontal disease, glaucoma, and hearing loss can all be detected early and can usually be treated or prevented.

The health history may be divided into seven parts: present health status; personal history; past health status; family history;

environmental health; nutritional history; and emotional self-assessment. A typical history might proceed like the following. It should be noted that each history has to be adapted to the individual client and questions not appropriate for that client deleted from the history.

PRESENT HEALTH STATUS
    I. Describe your present health.
        A. Is it better or worse than it was a year ago? five years ago?
        B. Have you any present concerns? (This helps the nurse to understand the value her client places on "health.")
    II. Current health statistics.
        A. Height and weight.
            1. What are your weight patterns over the last 5 to 10 years?
            2. If you diet, does your weight go up and down as you diet and stop dieting? (Obesity is a risk factor.)
        B. Immunization status (dates and any reactions).
            1. Tetanus-diptheria. (This is necessary every 10 years. Many deaths still occur from these causes.)
            2. Mumps. (This is a very serious disease in males and may cause sterility.)
            3. Rubella. (This is very serious for pregnant women in their first trimester and may cause birth defects in the fetus.)
            4 Polio. (Many young adults are not protected, or only incompletely so, by early vaccines.)
            5. Tuberculin skin test. (All young adults should have an annual tine test unless they have had a positive reaction, in which case the physician might order a chest x-ray.)
            6. Flu. (This is done at the discretion of the doctor; opinions differ.)
        C. Blood type and Rh factor.
        D. Allergies and types of reactions.
        E. Dates of last physical examination, physician/clinic, findings, advice and/or instructions.
        F. Date of last dental examination, dentist/clinic, findings, advice and/or instructions.
        G. Health and accident insurance. (Since many young and older adults have economic difficulty in providing adequate insurance, they may find it helpful to discuss the topic with the nurse.)
            1. Type.
            2. Conditions covered.

PERSONAL HISTORY
    I. Marital status or presence of significant other person. (This may indicate whether the client has someone to whom to turn for support in a crisis.)
    II. Religious preference. (This may have implications for medical intervention as, for example, with a Jehovah's Witness.)

III. Describe your "normal day," number of hours spent at work, home, etc. (This information will help the nurse understand the client's life-style.)
IV. Sleep patterns.
   A. Amount of sleep per night.
   B. Nap.
   C. Regularity of sleep patterns.
   D. Insomnia.
   E. Do you find you awaken more frequently than you used to?
V. Exercise
   A. Types and frequency of recreation: jogging, bicycling, swimming, dancing, tennis, skating, skiing, others.
   B. Types and frequency of daily activity: desk work, field farming, housekeeping, others.
VI. Physical fitness.
   A. Degree: poor, fair, excellent (refer to test, Page 23).
   B. Client's response to present state of physical fitness.
VII. Interests, hobbies, activities, recreation: amount of time devoted to each.
VIII. Driving.
   A. Miles driven per year.
   B. Wearing of seat belts: always, occasionally, never.
IX. Use of alcohol.
   A. Frequency and amounts: 41 or more drinks/week, 25-40, 7-24, 0-7.
   B. Type.
   C. Pattern over the last 5 to 10 years. If the use of alcohol seems excessive or if there is an indication that the use of alcohol may be problematic for the client, further assessment is needed.
   D. When you are anxious, do you reward yourself with a drink?
   E. Do you sometimes feel an urgent need for the first drink?
   F. Do you feel guilty about your drinking?
   G. Is it hard for you to talk about your drinking problem with anyone else?
   H. Have you ever been arrested for driving "under the influence"?
   I. Have you ever had a memory "blackout" after a night of heavy drinking?
   J. Has your drinking interfered with your work, your friends, or your family? If yes, how?
   K. Have you ever gone on a drinking binge?
   L. Check list for symptoms of alcoholism. Do you:
      1. Need a drink the "morning after"?
      2. Like to drink alone?
      3. Lose time from work due to drinking?
      4. Need a drink at a definite time daily?
      5. Have a loss of memory while or after drinking?
      6. Find yourself (or others) harder to get along with?
      7. Find your efficiency and ambition decreasing?
      8. Drink to relieve shyness, fear, or inadequacy?
      9. Find your drinking is harming or worrying your family?
      10. Find yourself more moody, jealous, or irritable after drinking?

If the answers are yes, the client is probably suffering from alcoholism. Recognition and acceptance of the disease is very important in the treatment of this disease.

X. Use of drugs: routine medications.
  A. Type.
  B. Quantity.
  C. Frequency.
XI. Safety.
  A. Occupational safety hazards.
  B. Safety factors in the home (see page 171).
XII. Traveling.
  A. Recent trips.
  B. Future trips.

The final topic in this category, sexual history, may be appropriately introduced now, or it may be discussed at any point at which the client wishes to raise it.

The nurse must take into account the possibility that the client may never have had previous experience giving information about his or her sexual behavior to a health care professional. The client may not understand either the reason for or the importance of this information. Consequently, it is imperative that the nurse choose wording that will neither offend nor alienate the client and that careful monitoring of nonverbal behavior serve as a guide to the way the interview proceeds. If the nurse could ask only one question in this area, it should be "Are there any questions you would like to ask me about sex?" Much ignorance prevails here and the nurse can often be of great help.

However, the nurse should be competent in both knowledge and skills of intervention in the area of human sexuality. For most nurses this will require preparation, specifically a course in human sexuality. The nurse must not only be able to assess this area as a part of the client's history, but also be prepared to answer the client's questions and to provide sexual counseling, when appropriate.

A sexual history is divided into four parts: family information; personal information; current data; and genital health.

XIII. Sexual history
  A. Family information
    1. Were your questions about sex answered freely, with embarrassment, evaded, or ignored?
    2. Who was most likely to speak about sex with you?
    3. How old were you when you learned about menstruation; wet dreams; sexual intercourse?
    4. From whom did you learn? How was the information explained?

      5. How demonstrative were your parents with each other?

      6. How demonstrative were your parents with you?

      7. What family member was most demonstrative with you?

B. Personal information

      1. What has been the greatest influence on your feelings about sex of any kind?

      2. How did you feel about sex play as a child?

      3. How old were you when you first engaged in sex play?

      4. What kinds of things did you do?

      5. How do you feel about masturbation?

      6. How often did you masturbate as a child?

      7. How old were you when you first masturbated?

      8. Where you ever punished for masturbation or sex play?

      9. Did you pet as an adolescent?

   10. What did petting include?

   11. When you petted did you feel worried about being caught?

   12. How old were you when you had sexual relations for the first time?

   13. Who was your first sex partner, and how did you feel about him (her)?

   14. What is your preference in terms of a sex partner or sexual activities?

   15. If you had premarital intercourse, how did you feel about it?

   16. How many sex partners have you had?

C. Current data

      1. Are you now having a sexual relationship with anyone?

      2. How would you describe it?

      3. How long have you been involved with your current major sex partner?

      4. How many sex partners have you had during the past year?

      5. How important is sex to you (not to your partner or to the relationship)?

      6. What do you like best about sex?

      7. What do you like least about sex?

      8. How often do you feel satisfied with sex?

      9. How often do you have sexual relations?

   10. How often does one of you want sex and the other does not?

   11. How often do you have sex when you don't want to, to please your partner?

   12. How often does your partner have sex just to please you?

   13. What causes you to become aroused?

   14. What causes your partner to become aroused?

   15. How often do you have a climax (orgasm) in sex relations?

   16. How often does your partner have orgasm?

   17. Are you satisfied with your climax?

   18. What kinds of things other than vaginal intercourse can excite you enough to reach a climax?

   19. What is your opinion about who should initiate sex?

20. Is it all right for you to initiate sex?
21. How comfortable are you and your partner about dressing and undressing in front of each other; touching genitals; rectal stimulation; rectal intercourse?
22. Do you and your partner talk about sex?
23. How does your sexual experience differ from what you thought it would be like before you had sex for the first time (or before you became sexually active)?
24. What would you like to change about your sex life?
25. Are there particular problems you would like to discuss?

D. Genital health
1. How do you protect yourself from being exposed to a sexually transmitted disease?
2. Have you ever experienced symptoms such as itching, pain or burning on urination, or slight discharge or unpleasant odor, which cleared up on their own? (If the answer is yes, obtain details of symptoms, self-treatment, etc.)
3. What symptoms would cause you to suspect that you might have a sexually transmitted disease?
4. Have you ever been treated for a sexually transmitted disease? (If the answer is yes, obtain details of symptoms, diagnosis, treatment, and follow-up.)

In addition to the four parts of the sexual history—family information, personal information, current data, and genital health—the following parts can be included for the adult having sexual problems.

E. Specific problems
1. Do you have trouble becoming sexually aroused?
Frequently   Occasionally, but not a problem   Never
2. If you frequently have trouble being aroused: (Describe)
   a. How often does this happen?
   b. When you are having difficulty, how long does it take you to eventually become aroused?
   c. Have you been aroused when interacting with another person?
   d. Have you been aroused from books, music, or daydreams (fantasy)?
   e. Do you fear pain? If yes, why?
3. Can you get an erection:
Always   Sometimes   Never
Often   Rarely   Not applicable
4. If you *rarely* or *never* get an erection:
   a. Have you ever been able to get an erection?
   b. Do you ever wake up with an erection?
   c. Can you get an erection by yourself? If yes, how?
5. If you have trouble *keeping* an erection, under what circumstances do you lose it?

6. Do you have pain with intercourse?
   Yes   No   Occasionally, but not a problem
7. If yes, you *do* have pain: (Describe)
   a. How often?
   b. When do you get it?
   c. Where is it located?
   d. How long have you had it?
   e. Does anything make it better?
   f. How long does it last?
8. Do you climax (achieve orgasm):
   Too soon   Later than you wish
   Never   Too seldom
9. If you climax too soon: (Describe)
   a. How long have you been aware of the problem?
   b. How long can you have intercourse before climaxing?
   c. How long do you *expect* to be able to have intercourse before climaxing?
   d. What have you tried to delay it?
   e. Is it getting worse?
   f. What is your partner's reaction?
10. If your climax takes too long; (Describe)
    a. How long have you been aware of the problem?
    b. How long does it take you to climax?
    c. What have you tried to speed it up?
    d. Is it getting worse?
    e. How long can your partner have intercourse before climax?
    f. Does your partner know about your problem? What is his or her reaction?
11. Do you climax:
    a. From masturbation.   Yes   No   Sometimes
    b. From partner's mouth or
       hand stimulation.   Yes   No   Sometimes
    c. From vaginal intercourse.   Yes   No   Sometimes
12. If no to any of the above questions:
    a. Have you tried to climax
       that way?   Yes   No
    b. Have you ever climaxed that
       way?   Yes   No
    c. Did you formerly climax that
       way but no longer can?   Yes   No
13. If you have never experienced climax (orgasm), what do you think is the reason for that?
14. Do you have diabetes, heart trouble, or high blood pressure? Does anyone in your family?
15. Do you take any drugs, including uppers, downers, marijuana, or prescribed medications? (List them.)
16. On the average, what volume of alcoholic beverages do you drink in a week?
17. Have you had any major surgery?

Since the cessation of menstruation is a major milestone for women, nurses should obtain information specifically about the event. The following interview schedule was adapted from a longer questionaire designed to obtain normative data about how women experience menopause. After the first four questions, the interview schedule is divided into sections for premenopausal, menopausal, and postmenopausal women respectively.

F. Female Menopause
   1. How old was your mother when she experienced menopause?
   2. How did your mother describe her experience of menopause to you?
   3. Have you had the number of children you wanted?
      ____ Yes
      ____ No, would rather have had _____
   4. What conception control measures are you using?
      ____ Abstinence   ____ Hysterectomy
      ____ I.U.D.   ____ Condom
      ____ Birth control pills ____ Vasectomy
      ____ Diaphragm   ____ Tubes tied
      ____ Rhythm   ____ None
      ____ Foam   Other: _____

   For premenopausal women only
   5. *When* do you expect to begin to experience menopausal symptoms and *why*?
   6. *What* do you expect will happen to you during menopause and *why*?
   7. How would you describe your feelings as you approach menopause?

   For menopausal women only
   8. How old were you when menopausal symptoms began?
   9. What symptoms have you experienced and how severe are they? (Use a scale of 0=none; 1=slight; 2-moderate; and 3-marked.)

Symptoms	Severity
Hot flashes	____
Drenching perspiration	____
Tingling	____
Palpitations	____
Frequency or urgency voiding	____
Vaginitis	____
Painful intercourse	____
Depression	____
Back pain	____
Tension	____
Bad dreams	____
Fatigue	____

Increased nervousness   ——

Headaches   ——

Insomnia   ——

Irritability   ——

Dizziness   ——

Other: _____   ——

10. Are you on any medication specifically for menopausal symptoms?

____ Yes   ____ No

11. Are you on any other medications?

____ Yes   ____ No

12. Are you concerned or inconvenienced by any menopausal symptoms which you have not discussed with your doctor?

____ Yes   ____ No

If yes, *what* are they and *why* have you not discussed them with your doctor?

13. Describe your present menstrual cycles, if any.

14. How do you cope with the changes which your body is currently undergoing?

15. How would you describe your feelings as you are experiencing menopause?

16. Compared with women you know, how would you rate yourself?

____ Having an easier time with menopause than most

____ About the same as other women

____ Having a harder time with menopause than most

Do you have an explanation for this?

For postmenopausal women only

17. How old were you when menstruation completely stopped?

18. Are you currently on hormone replacement therapy?

____ Yes   ____ No

If yes, what are you taking?

19. Are you currently experiencing any symptoms which you attribute to having reached menopause?

____ Yes   ____ No

20. In retrospect, how would you describe your feelings about menopause?

21. What impact has menopause had upon your life?

Although the signs of male menopause are more generalized, the nurse should include assessment in this area and encourage the client to discuss his feelings and perceptions.

G. Male Menopause

1. What symptoms have you experienced and how severe are they? (Use a scale of 0=none; 1=slight; 2=moderate; and 3=marked.)

Symptoms	*Severity*
Hot flashes	____
Sweating attacks	____
Anxiety	____
Depression	____
Forgetfulness	____
Nightmares	____
Worry	____
Impatience	____
Moodiness	____
Touchiness	____

2. How old were you when symptoms began?
3. Are you on any medication specifically for symptoms?
   ____ Yes   ____ No
   If yes, what are you taking?
4. Are you concerned or inconvenienced by any menopausal symptoms which you have not discussed with your doctor?
   ____ Yes   ____ No
5. How do you cope with the changes which your body is currently undergoing?
6. How would you describe your feelings as you are experiencing menopause?
7. Compared with men you know, how would you rate yourself?
   ____ Having an easier time with menopause than most
   ____ About the same as other men
   ____ Having a harder time with menopause than most
   Do you have an explanation for this?

The ability to offer older adults an opportunity to discuss possible areas of concern related to their sexual behavior depends heavily on the interviewer's choice of words. Many older adults would not understand the meaning of the question "Are you sexually active?" The interviewer conveys a more clear meaning with "Do you and your wife (husband) (partner) still have sex?"; or "Do you and your wife (husband) (partner) still make love?" It is impossible to predict in advance whether the clients will experience a sense of relief at being allowed to be candid, a sense of outrage at a perceived invasion of privacy, or a sense of the ridiculous because that part of their lives ceased long ago. The unpredictability of the response is not sufficient reason for avoiding the issue.

Nurses should use their common sense about the extent of the sex history they take from the older adult. There is little point in inquiring about the source of their sex education or the occasion of their first menstrual period. Such information may not even be open to accurate recall and will be much less helpful than a thorough review of the present and the more recent past. Nurses can judge what they need to pursue depending on the unique situation of each client. The most important thing to remember is to avoid making assumptions based on appearance only.

This is a rather formidable list of questions, and it is not essential that the nurse secure answers to all of them at the first meeting, certainly not in writing, which may tend to make the client even more nervous. It is essential that the nurse first establish herself as someone with whom the client may talk freely and confidently on this important topic.

PAST HEALTH STATUS
I. Record of childhood and adult diseases, illnesses, injuries, and recoveries.
II. Emotional problems.
III. General level of health. (Make sure to note any serious or chronic diseases.)
IV. Hospitalizations or surgery: organs repaired or removed, x-rays taken, medication.
V. Menstrual history (onset, days in cycle, duration, date of last period, discomfort).
VI. Obstetric history.
   A. Complete pregnancies.
   B. Incomplete pregnancies: duration, termination, circumstances.
   C. Spontaneous or induced abortion.
   D. Stillbirth.
   E. Children with defects, anomalies, metabolic disorders, etc.

FAMILY HISTORY
I. Genetic disabilities in extended family.
II. Tendencies to conditions or diseases in family: heart disease, cancer, diabetes, epilepsy, arthritis, hearing defects, hypertension, mental retardation illness, visual defects, TB.
III. Family habits that may lead to health problems: overeating, drinking.
IV. Family members, including maternal/paternal grandparents, siblings of parents, and their children. (Draw a family tree and include ages, whether living or deceased, cause of death, level of health, evidence of serious or chronic illness; see Figure 16-1.)

This area is of great importance in determining the risk factors of the client. Young adults frequently do not think much about the genetic influence in terms of risk factors on their own lives, nor do they stop to realize what good prospects of success they have in avoiding or minimizing these risks if the situation is considered early.

Risk factors — cancer
A. Is there a history of cancer in your family?

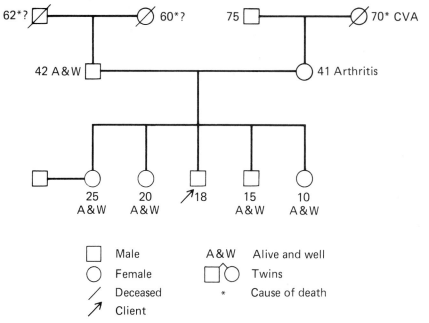

FIGURE 16-1 List siblings in birth order, oldest on the left. The horizontal line (—) indicates the marital relationship, with the male symbol to the left. The vertical line (|) indicates offspring.

B. Do you smoke?
   If yes, how much, how long, and do you inhale the smoke?
   Do you smoke a pipe, cigar, or cigarettes?

C. Do you eat foods high in fat? Foods low in fiber? Foods high in nitrates?

D. Do you drink distilled alcohol regularly? How many drinks per week?

E. Did you ever receive radiation for tonsilitis or an enlarged thymus gland?

F. Do you know the seven warning signs of cancer?

G. For women only:
   1. Are you presently taking estrogen for the discomforts of menopause?
   2. Do you do the monthly self-breast exam?
   3. Did your mother ever take a synthetic estrogen diethylstilbestrol (DES) early in her pregnancy?

Risk factors — heart disease

H. Is there a history of hypertension or heart disease, particularly before the age of 60?

I. Are you hypertensive? Is your hypertension being treated?

J.   How would you describe yourself in terms of the following behaviors?

Always   Occasionally   Never

Over-ambitious
Highly motivated
Constantly on the go
Feeling pressure at home
Feeling pressure at work

Environmental health is a very important topic. The information
about the clients' home will help the nurse determine a feeling for
their life-style, and information about possible pollution will not
only inform the nurse but may alert the clients themselves to un-
suspected dangers. Smoking is a risk factor for both heart disease
and cancer. It is to be noted, moreover, that it affects the health
of other members of the family as well as that of the smoker. Respiratory infections are more frequent in the children of smokers
than in those of nonsmokers. Young adults are particularly liable
to resort to tobacco to cope with stress without realizing the implications in terms of health.

ENVIRONMENTAL HEALTH
  I. Home environment.
      A. Do you own or rent your home?
      B. How would you describe the appearance of your house? Neighbor-
          hood? Community?
      C. How many members are there in your household?
      D. Is emergency transportation available?
      E. Are health care facilities accessible?
  II. Environmental danger.
      A. Air pollution.
          1. Do you know of any air pollution in your neighborhood?
          2. How close are you to the nearest factory, heavily traveled street,
              and electric power plant?
          3. How do you rank your work environment in terms of pollution?
          4. Are you regularly exposed to factory smoke, herbicides, etc.?
          5. Do you come into contact with asbestos in your line of work?
          6. Do you use aerosol sprays, hair sprays, or insect repellants?
          7. Do you smoke? If yes, give amount in packs, pipesful, or cigars
              per day; type; habit patterns over the last 5 to 10 years.

Smoking, specifically the patterns and factors of smoking, should
be further evaluated.

          8. How much tar and nicotine does your brand of cigarettes have?
          9. Do you smoke your cigarette all the way down?

10. Do you inhale your cigarette, pipe, or cigar smoke?
11. Do or did your parents smoke?
12. Do other members in your household smoke?
13. Do you enjoy smoking *with* other people?
14. Do you smoke to relax?
15. Do you smoke automatically — that is are you sometimes not aware that you have lit a cigarette?
16. When do you smoke?

What time of day?	During what activity?	How many?

B. Noise pollution.
   1. Are you aware of any regular noise pollution in your home or work environment?
   2. Do you ride the subway?
   3. Do you ride a motorcycle?
   4. Do you drive a snowmobile or motor boat?
   5. Do you regularly listen to loud music?

C. Water pollution.
   1. Do you use city water? Have your own well?
   2. Is your water soft? Do you use a water softener?
   3. Are you aware of any water pollution in your environment, such as agricultural run-off, road salt, sewage, or chemical pollution?
   4. Are you pleased with the taste, smell, and appearance of the water you drink?
   5. Do you wash or peel fruits and vegetables before eating?
   6. Are you able to grow any of your own food?

D. Radiation hazard.
   1. How many x-rays have you had in the past year?
   2. Do you keep a record of the number and type of x-rays you have?
   3. Do you have routine dental x-rays?
   4. Do you sunbathe?
   5. Do you wear a hat or use suntan lotion in the sun?

NUTRITIONAL HISTORY

Before the meeting with the nurse the client should fill out a record of all food taken in a 24-hour period, and perhaps mail it in. (See Table 18-1.)

The nurse should then analyze the diet for caloric intake, including the comparison with the suggested caloric intake for comparable heights and weights.

TABLE 18-1 24-hour food recall

	Food	Quantity	Calories
Breakfast			
Lunch			
Dinner			
Total			

Based on the information supplied by the client in the 24-hour recall (Table 18-1) the nurse should analyze the diet in terms of food groups and basic nutrients. The format shown in Table 18-2 may be helpful in doing the diet analysis.

TABLE 18-2 24-hour nutritional recall analysis

	Foods & Amt.	Cal.	Food Groups					Vitamins & Minerals						Iron	Calcium	Protein	Fats	Carbohydrates
			Meat	Milk	Veg.	Bread	Misc.	Vit. A	Vit. D	Vit. C	Vit. E	Vit B$_1$	Vit. B$_2$	Iron	Calcium	Protein	Fats	Carbohydrates
Breakfast																		
Lunch																		
Dinner																		
Total																		

I. Analysis
   Food Group

      Meat – 2 servings per day
      Milk – 2 servings per day
      Vegetable and Fruit – 4 servings per day
      Bread – 4 servings per day
      Meat Group – Meat, Fish, Poultry, and Eggs
         – 3 oz. = 1 serving
         – 2 eggs = 1 serving
         – 1 cup cooked beans = 1 serving
         – 4 tbsp. peanut butter = 1 serving
      Milk Group – Milk, Cheese, Ice Cream
         – 1 cup = 1 serving
         – 1 oz. cheese = 1 serving
      Vegetable and Fruit Group
         – ½ cup vegetable or fruit = 1 serving
      Bread and Cereal Group
         – 1 slice bread = 1 serving

– 5 saltines = 1 serving
– ½ to ¾ cup cooked cereal = 1 serving
– ½ to ¾ cup cooked pasta = 1 serving
Vitamins and Minerals

Refer to a nutrition textbook for the recommended daily allowances for vitamins and minerals.

When the nurse meets with the client to discuss these results she can secure answers to the following questions:

1 Describe your present appetite.
2 Do you take any daily vitamin or mineral supplement?
3 What are your favorite foods?
4 Do you have any food dislikes? Allergies?
5 Do you hold any religious beliefs which influence your diet?
6 Who prepares your food?
7 How often do you eat in restaurants?
8 What is your weekly food budget?
9 What kinds of convenience foods do you eat?
10 Do you use iodized salt?
11 Do you wear dentures? Is chewing a problem for you?
12 Do you ever have problems with heartburn? Constipation? Belching?

II. Weight control
  A. Are or were your parents obese? One of them? Both of them?
  B. Were you "overweight" as a child?
  C. For women:
    1. Did you put on weight with any of your pregnancies? Was the most significant weight gain with your first pregnancy?
    2. Did you put on weight during menopause?

TABLE 18-3 Daily caloric requirements for levels of activity

	Men cal/lb. body wt.	Women cal/lb. body wt.
Sedentary	16	14
Light	17	16
Moderate	21	18
Active	26	22

Sedentary: Includes occupations that involve sitting most of the day, such as secretarial work and studying.
Light: Includes activities that involve standing most of the day, such as teaching or laboratory work.
Moderate: Includes walking, gardening, and housework.
Active: Includes dancing, skating, and manual labor such as farm work or construction.

    D. Do you eat rapidly?
    E. Do you keep food "out in plain sight"?
    F. Do you eat when you're upset?
    G. Are you feeling lonely, embarrassed, or depressed about your obesity?
    H. What rooms other than the kitchen do you eat in?
    I. Do you shop with a list?
    J. Do you shop on an empty stomach?
    K. Do you measure your food when you're on a diet?
    L. Do the people you live with help you and praise you for losing weight?
    M. Do you let yourself get overtired?
    N. Do you leave food on your plate?
    O. When eating, do you usually take "seconds"?

For clients with weight problems, Table 18-4 may be helpful. By keeping track of a typical day's eating habits, the client can better pin-point trouble spots.

TABLE 18-4 Food diary

What time you ate	What food you ate	Where and what you were doing	Were you alone?	How did you feel?

III. Food Budget
    A. Do you own a refrigerator, stove, and/or freezer?
    B. How do you travel to and from the store?
    C. What kind of companionship do you have at meal times?
    D. Do you shop with a shopping list?
    E. How much money do you spend on food each week?

The nurse can suggest that clients on a budget use Table 18-5 as a guide while doing their shopping.

TABLE 18-5   Bargains in the basic four food groups*

Food Group	Usually Less Expensive, More Food Value for the Money	Usually More Expensive, Less Food Value for the Money
Milk products	Concentrated, fluid, and dry nonfat milk, evaporated, buttermilk	Fluid whole milk, chocolate drink, condensed milk, sweet or sour cream
	Mild cheddar, Swiss, cottage cheese	Sharp cheddar, Roquefort or blue; grated or sliced cheese, cream cheese, yogurt
	Ice milk, imitation ice milk, imitation ice cream	Ice cream, sherbet
Meats and meat substitutes		
Meat	Good and standard grades	Prime and choice grades
	Less tender cuts	Tender cuts
	Home-cooked meats	Canned meats, sliced luncheon meats
	Pork or beef liver, heart, kidney, tongue	Calf liver
Poultry	Stewing chickens, whole broiler-fryers, large turkeys	Poultry parts, specialty products, canned poultry, small turkeys
Fish	Rock cod, butterfish, other fresh fish in season, frozen filets, steaks, and sticks	Salmon, crab, lobster, prawns, shrimp, oysters
Eggs	Grade A	Grade AA
Beans, peas, and lentils	Dried beans, peas, lentils	Canned baked beans, soups
Nuts	Peanut butter, walnuts, other nuts in shell	Pecans, cashews, shelled nuts, prepared nuts

TABLE 18-5   Bargains in the basic four food groups (contd.)

Vegetables, fruits	Local vegetables and fruits in season	Out-of-season vegetables and fruits, unusual vegetables and fruits, those in short supply
Vitamin-A rich	Carrots, collards, sweet potatoes, green leafy vegetables, spinach, pumpkin, winter squash, broccoli, and in-season cantaloupe, apricots, persimmons	Tomatoes, Brussels sprouts, asparagus, peaches, watermelon, papaya, bananas, tangerines
Vitamin-C rich	Oranges, grapefruit, and their juice, cabbage, greens, green pepper, cantaloupe, strawberries, tomatoes, broccoli in season	Tangerines, apples, bananas, peaches, pears
Others	Medium-sized potatoes, nonbaking types	Baking potatoes, new potatoes, canned or frozen potatoes, potato chips
	Romaine, leaf lettuce	Iceberg lettuce, frozen specialty packs of vegetables
Breads, cereals	Whole wheat and enriched flour	Stone-ground, unenriched, and cake flour
	Whole grain and enriched breads	French, Vienna, other specialty breads, hard rolls
	Homemade rolls and coffee cake	Ready-made rolls and coffee cakes, frozen or partially baked products
	Whole grain or restored uncooked cereals	Ready-to-eat cereals, puffed, sugar-coated
	Graham crackers, whole grain wafers	Zwieback, specialty crackers, and wafers
	Enriched uncooked macaroni, spaghetti, noodles	Unenriched, canned, or frozen macaroni, spaghetti, noodles
	Brown rice, converted rice	Quick-cooking, seasoned, or canned rice

*Source: Cook, F., C. Groppe, and M. Ferree: *Balanced food values and cents*, University of California Agricultural Extension Service, Pub. HXT-42, Berkeley, Calif., 1970, pp. 6–7.

EMOTIONAL SELF-ASSESSMENT
"Relative" here again should be stressed. It is not a matter of good or bad, black or white; it is a matter of relative achievement in these tasks, and the client can be encouraged to continue to grow and develop.

I. Developmental tasks
   A. Young adult.
      1. Establish independence from one's parents.
      2. Develop one's own sense of values.
      3. Develop a sense of personal identity.
      4. Form intimate relationships with people outside the family.
   B. Middle adult.
      1. Separate from parents and children by becoming independent.
      2. Increase self-esteem through self-awareness.
      3. Review one's value system.
      4. Prepare for the future.
   C. Older adult.
      1. Recognize that aging can be a positive experience.
      2. Make adjustments and redefine physical and social space.
      3. Maintain feelings of self-worth, pride, and usefulness.
      4. Strive toward developing a personal set of goals as one prepares for death.
II. Emotional changes. (Describe briefly.)
   A. Psychological self (e.g., disappointed at work, difficulty at school).
   B. Physical self (e.g., gained weight, glasses).
   C. Beliefs, values, and expectations (e.g., changed religious affiliation, new sexual behaviors).
   D. Relevant social network (e.g., divorce, marriage and new baby).
   E. Nonhuman environment (e.g., move to new apartment, house).
III. Using the Holmes Scale of Life Events (see page 5), calculate your score.
   A. High potential for health crisis: over 300.
   B. Moderate potential for health crisis: 150–300.
   C. Low potential for health crisis: under 150.
IV. Describe your greatest personal strengths.
V. Describe your greatest personal limitations.
VI. Describe briefly how you cope with stress, giving an example of an extreme situation which increased your awareness of your ability to cope.
VII. Preretirement preparations.
   A. Are you considering retiring? When?
   B. Have you begun to plan for living arrangements after retirement?
   C. Have you considered a retirement career, business, or self-employment after retirement?
   D. What hobbies do you have? Outside interests?
   E. Briefly describe how you spend your leisure time.

     F. What provisions have you made for your health care after retirement?

     G. Are you aware of your social security benefits?

     H. Have you calculated your income after retirement?

     I. Is there a preretirement program at work or available for you to attend?

Dental, vision, and hearing examinations are to be included in this general assessment. The nurse or physician should include a routine dental, vision, and hearing check; the private dentist, ophthalmologist or optometrist, and audiologist should provide the full examination.

EYE EXAMINATION

Adults who wear glasses need an eye examination annually. For others, every other year is sufficient.

     The nurse will have an opportunity to discuss some popular myths about vision. Contrary to popular belief, eyes cannot be damaged by use, even excessive use for fine work or in poor light. There is no such thing as eye strain. We can no more strain our eyes from too much looking than we can strain our noses from too much smelling. Eye fatigue can result from the action of accommodation or convergence of muscles, but it is relieved by rest and does no permanent damage, nor does sitting close to a TV or reading a book up close. Another myth is that eye exercises are an alternative to glasses, and a third is that a delay in getting reading glasses will preserve vision.[2]

     If clients have no professional who provides vision care, the nurse might review for them the training, functions, differences, and similarities among ophthalmologists, optometrists, and opticians.[3] It is important for the nurse to obtain vision information in the family history, for an inherited tendency to certain problems does exist. As Perkins suggests,

> There is now overwhelming evidence that the siblings and children of patients with both chronic simple and closed glaucoma show a higher incidence of the disease than the rest of the population.[4]

HEARING EXAMINATION

If they are not conscious of problems, adults may feel they do not need a hearing test. But it is important for them to have one annually, and basic audiometric tests can be given by the nurse. Progressive hearing loss can occur from exposure to certain types of noise (see Chapter V). If a client is a tree surgeon, for instance, the nurse should inquire if he has ear protectors, and if he wears them at work. Neglecting to wear ear protectors is a common and dangerous practice of many adults.[5]

     Hearing loss can also occur with age, due to vascular insufficiency of the cochlear organ. Studies show that smokers demonstrate greater hearing loss than others. Smoking reduces the blood supply by vasospasm induced by nicotine, by atherosclerotic narrowing of vessels, and by thrombotic occlusions.[6]

DENTAL EXAMINATION

Young adults have a very high incidence of gum diseases, higher even than that of tooth diseases. Routine dental cleaning and examination are essential at least once a year, but are preferable every 6 months. This is extremely important in preventing the development of serious dental problems in the middle years. Even well-educated young adults do not know that the loss of teeth with aging is not inevitable. Though every middle or older adult in the family may wear dentures, there is no reason why the young adult must anticipate the same for himself. Certainly there is an inherited trend; but the determining factor is often the degree and extent of routine dental care and dental hygiene. There is another very strong motive for care of the teeth at this age which the nurse should emphasize: the loss of teeth in itself accelerates aging and is often the cause of gastrointestinal problems in old age.

The nurse can check the mouth for plaque and inquire into the clients' daily dental habits. It is not necessary to use toothpaste every time they brush their teeth, or to use toothpaste at all. The object of brushing is to remove plaque from the teeth, which is done by the friction of the toothbrush (a soft-bristled brush should be used), and to remove food particles. Dental floss is indispensable for the latter purpose, since it reaches the space between the teeth where food is retained. The sooner after eating the teeth are brushed, the better. It is now possible to buy toothbrushes in carrying cases, so that they can be used after every meal. Many techniques of cleaning the teeth are now available: blotting, daily cleansing of the gums and spaces around teeth, has become a respected and popular method. The client should, of course, follow his dentist's advice.

When clients complete the total health assessment, they should know more about themselves than they did before, strengths as well as weaknesses. Based on the total health assessment the nurse can begin developing a health maintenance plan with the client. Goals related to teaching can be identified, with the nurse providing up-to-date medical information to help the client arrive at his own decisions.

BIBLIOGRAPHY

1. *Nutrition in Pregnancy-Care of the Pregnant Patient*, dev. by The University of Southern California School of Medicine, Raritan, N. J., Omni, Ortho Pharmaceutical Corp., 1974.
2. Reedshaw, G.: "Ophthalmic Old Wives' Tales," *Med. J. Australia*, 2:337-339, 1973.
3. Shaver, David V.: "Opticianry, Optometry, and Ophthalmology: An Overview," *Nursing Digest*, 3 no. (5):54-57, 1975.
4. Perkins, E. S.: "Screening for Ophthalmic Conditions," *Practitioner*, 211: 171-177, 1973.
5. Sataloff, J., et al.: "Hearing Conservation," *Industrial Med. Surg.*, 42:23-26, 1973.
6. Zelman, S.: "Correlation of Smoking History with Hearing Loss," *J. Amer. Med. Assoc.*, 23:920, 1973.

Index

Venereal diseases, 66
Vertebral compression, 84
Vision loss of elderly, 155
   driving and, 172
Vitamin deficiencies, 177–178
Vitamins, 38
Vomiting during pregnancy, 47

Walking, 98–99, 169
Water pollution, 76–77
Water softeners, 77
Weight reduction by elderly, 176
Widowhood, 158, 207
   sexual activity and, 130

Women: changing social roles of, 3
   increased opportunities for, 7

X-rays: cancer and, 87–88
   radiation hazards from, 78

Young adults: developmental tasks of,
   9–12
   hazardous activities of, 32–34
   nutrition for, 37–49
   sexuality of, 51–67

Zen macrobiotic diet, 43–44